THE
Slightly
GREENER
METHOD

DETOXIFYING YOUR HOME IS EASIER, FASTER, AND LESS EXPENSIVE THAN YOU THINK

TONYA HARRIS, MSHN, BCHN®

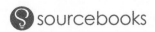

sourcebooks

Published by Sourcebooks
P.O. Box 4410, Naperville, Illinois 60567-4410
(630) 961-3900
sourcebooks.com

Library of Congress Cataloging-in-Publication Data

Names: Harris, Tonya, author.
Title: The slightly greener method : detoxifying your home is easier,
    faster, and less expensive than you think / Tonya Harris, MSHN BCHN.
Description: Naperville, Illinois : Sourcebooks, [2021] | Includes
    bibliographical references and index.
Identifiers: LCCN 2021001188 (print) | LCCN 2021001189 (ebook)
Subjects: LCSH: Toxins--Physiological effect. | Detoxification (Health)
Classification: LCC RA1250 .H37 2021 (print) | LCC RA1250 (ebook) | DDC
    613--dc23
LC record available at https://lccn.loc.gov/2021001188
LC ebook record available at https://lccn.loc.gov/2021001189

Printed and bound in the United States of America.
VP 10 9 8 7 6 5 4 3 2 1

For James, Eric, Kaylee, and Lyndsey.
Thank you for your love, support, and encouragement,
and for letting me share your stories.

Contents

Part IV: Slightly Greener Cleaning   195

Author's Note

The Slightly Greener Method was created to help families develop a plan for detoxifying their homes by making small changes over time. I wanted to create a blueprint to make it easier to know where to start and to avoid the overwhelming feelings we so often face when starting out on this healthier, less-toxic journey.

It's been developed through years of research from my own experience, getting my master's degree, and client work, and it was then refined many times to help you discover which toxins to prioritize avoiding for your unique needs, since we can't avoid them all. It's the system I would have wanted when I first started out in 2006, when I felt the need to toss everything, driving my family (and myself!) crazy.

This method revolves around three main areas of the home: the kitchen (foods and beverages), bathroom (personal care products and cosmetics), and cleaning products. I believe that reducing toxins in these three areas of your home will result in the biggest changes in your toxic exposure. As you move through each area of your home and the process becomes easier, move on to the next section. Keep coming back to this book and use it as a resource, or do the method again as things change.

While you're reading this book, please keep in mind that removing toxins is just one part of a healthier lifestyle. While I believe the toxins that may be lurking in what we eat, the products we use to get ready, and the air we breathe in our homes are often a huge missing piece of the puzzle when it comes to health, it's also important to remember that being under the care of a licensed medical professional is important. The information in this book is not meant to diagnose or treat any medical conditions. Always discuss any health concerns with your doctor, and do not go off any medications without speaking to your licensed medical professional first.

Throughout this book, you will also see resources and safer brands that I recommend. Because links and product ingredients change often, be sure to visit this book's website at slightlygreener-book.com. There, you will find updated information, downloadable cheat sheets, and a current list of resources and brands.

And now, let's dig in and begin those first steps to a healthier home!

Part I

The Challenge of Detoxifying Our Homes

1

Why *Slightly* Greener

You've probably seen headlines like "Toxins Are All Around Us" on the news or in your Facebook feed. Although most of those articles are clickbait backed by dubious science, their underlying message is true. Our modern world is filled with more harmful substances than ever before. But the good news is that making small changes to become slightly greener can make you and your family significantly healthier.

"Do the best you can until you know better. Then when you know better, do better."

This Maya Angelou quote distills the essence of the Slightly Greener Method. I repeat it often when I teach clients how to reduce their toxin exposure, showing them how harmful chemicals can be found in nearly every product they bring into their homes, which is often quite shocking for them. "Doing better" refers to becoming *slightly greener* once you know how. It means making small changes—slowly over time—to avoid toxins in the foods you eat, the personal care products you use, and the cleaning products you buy. Notice Ms. Angelou didn't say, "Be perfect!" She also didn't say, "Shame on you for not knowing earlier!"

When I meet someone new and explain that I teach people how to eliminate toxins for a living, they stare back at me with wide eyes. I see their fear and the thoughts racing through their mind: *Please don't tell me I can give my kids cancer by feeding them hot dogs.* But once I explain that small changes over time can drastically reduce *overall toxin exposure*, their face softens. Then I add, "Sticking with those changes, even for just a few days, can have a tremendous impact on your health." Now they are hanging on my every word. I go on to explain that the approach I've developed to reduce toxin exposure, the Slightly Greener Method, is simple, inexpensive, fun, and doesn't require being a domestic diva. Then they smile. At this point, I've earned a new client or a made new friend—usually both.

Toxins lurk in much of the food we feed children, as well as in personal care products like shampoo, soap, and toothpaste—even ones labeled for babies and toddlers. These chemicals can affect every aspect of kids' health and wellness, including learning and behavior. In this book, I will teach you easy tips and tricks for making your home slightly greener—and your family significantly healthier—in ways that will transform your life. You'll also be a bit horrified at what you learn, all the sneaky and deceptive ways toxins have crept into your home, your food, and the very air you breathe. You might scream, pull your hair out, or hurl this book so hard against the wall that the windowpanes shake. It's OK.

After reading this book, you won't wake up and magically have a fully detoxified, chemical-free home. You can't blink and make all the harmful toxins disappear. However, you will be more educated. And with your new knowledge, you can make small, impactful changes. With each one, you'll feel healthier. As you stick with them, you'll feel lighter and calmer too.

When my clients first learn about how much gnarly stuff they've been shoveling into their mouths and slathering on their skin, they get uncomfortable—and they feel guilty.

Oh no, they think. *I've been pouring chemicals all over my kids. On their skin! In their mouths! (And in mine.)* I remind them of Maya Angelou's words: "When you know better, do better." If you learn anything from this book, it's that guilt can be just as toxic as hidden chemicals. I empower my clients to take back control. And I don't allow them to listen to the inner voice that says, "How could you?"

You didn't know. I didn't either.

But now we do.

Rule number one of the Slightly Greener Method? No guilt allowed!

On my dresser at home, I have a photo of my son Eric on his first birthday. He's sitting in his high chair, all adorable with chubby cheeks, drool on his chin. In that image, he's holding a fistful of birthday cake, preparing to cram it into his mouth. Right there on his high chair, in huge letters across the plastic tray smothered with icing and cake, it reads: MICROBAN. I bought that particular high chair because it was made of antibacterial plastic. "No germs getting in *this* baby's mouth!" I said. It was 1999, and back then, I had no idea that Microban is a brand name for triclosan, an endocrine disruptor. You'll learn all about endocrine disruptors, the nasty health problems they cause, and how to avoid them in this book. Back then, I didn't know. Eric wasn't eating many germs, but boy was he was shoveling harmful endocrine disruptors into his mouth by the handful! *Do the best you can until you know better.* As human beings, and especially as parents, most of us do what we think is right. We believe that "someone" out there will prevent us from bringing harmful substances into our homes. Sadly, that person doesn't exist. Many new parents think, *No one would put dangerous chemicals in baby products, right?*

Wrong.

Before I became an environmental toxin expert, I assumed someone else was "taking care of it." Health food company CEOs? The FDA? What about pediatricians? They're alerting parents about the dangers they need to know about, right? Although doctors provide valuable, life-saving expertise, protecting us from dangerous chemicals in consumer products isn't always a service they provide. When was the last time your doctor said, "Hmm, your son is having attention issues. What kind of toothpaste does he use?" Or, "Does he consume foods that contain a lot of artificial colors?" There aren't always screening questions at the pediatrician's office for environmental toxins—at least not yet.

For the past five years, my business, Slightly Greener, has filled the void that most people—especially parents—need. I teach micro changes and habits for reducing toxins in your home without wrecking your budget, your relationships, or even your day. The key is starting small, sticking with it, and building from there. Ask anyone who knows me. "I can't cook," I say, "but I can whip up twenty-two chap sticks in four minutes." If I can do it, so can you. I grew up in a small town in the Midwest, just outside Chicago. People from my hometown wave to one another, work hard, and enjoy life to the fullest. I apply that same Midwestern sensibility to the Slightly Greener lifestyle. You don't have to sacrifice happiness to be healthy. I won't ask you to throw away that giant bag of Cheetos in your pantry.

If you remove all the fun from life (an occasional scoop of bright blue ice cream or spritz of your favorite perfume), then it's no longer *living*. But if you can buy or make healthy products 80 percent of the time, you can still eat hot dogs occasionally. You don't have to exist on blades of grass (organic, of course!) and tree bark, I promise. I'll show you how to pick and choose which products to allow in your fridge, your pantry, your medicine cabinet, and under your sink. Together, we'll toss out the most harmful products in your home. The Slightly Greener Method is like decluttering with an added health boost. *Goodbye, chemicals. Hello, health and organization.*

Genetics, nutritional status, and general overall health can also play powerful roles in how our bodies handle chemicals. Our general health impacts how and when we will feel the effects of toxins. If you're in good health overall, you're in a better position to process and eliminate harmful chemicals. Illness—even as mild as a cold—can decrease your tolerance to household chemicals. Stress can also affect the body's ability to handle and process toxic chemicals. I always tell clients: implement just a few small changes at a time—whichever ones feel easiest for you—*and* take extra good care of your health. With those two adjustments, your home (and *you*) will be healthier overall.

Over time, the small changes I suggest become habits. It becomes so easy—practically automatic—to stick with it. And the benefits are huge.

What *are* toxins, really?

First, let's clear up any confusion about the definition of *toxins*. We hear the word *toxin* a lot, but few people truly understand its meaning. You might be surprised to learn that most people misuse the term. A toxin is a natural poison from a biological source, like a plant or an animal, such as the venom from a poisonous snake. A *toxicant* is an artificial substance introduced into the environment, like lead paint or formaldehyde. Both are harmful to the body, but toxins occur naturally in the environment, while toxicants are human made. The confusion arises because most people who aren't scientists *say* toxin, but what they *mean* is toxicant. I use the word *toxin* myself because I think it sounds more approachable than toxicant, which sounds scientific and scary. In this book, I will use the word *toxin* when I refer to artificial substances, because it's what we're used to hearing and because I like to remove the scare factor as much as possible.

Toxins cause harm in the body, and they can affect just about every biological system: neurological, respiratory, and endocrine, to name a few. Toxins are sneaky. They can creep into our homes in so many hidden ways. Just about everything we own contains toxins: furniture, electronics, pool toys, even toothpaste. Toxins can hide in flooring, food, cleaning products...the list goes on.[1] The good news?

You don't have to get rid of them all to have a measurable effect on your health.

How do toxins get into our products?

Despite the fact that an overwhelming number of consumer products contain toxins, companies can slap a "natural" or "safe" label on pretty much anything. You read that right: any old product they please. Terms like *natural* aren't regulated, so it's perfectly legal to throw a meaningless "natural" or "dermatologist approved" label on any product and start shipping it out via Amazon to mailboxes everywhere.

Remember the story of Goliath, the giant Philistine warrior who was defeated by David, the scrawny underdog? Consumers, people like you and me, are the little guy in this scenario. Most of the items we use in our homes are manufactured by multinational companies with Goliath-sized marketing budgets. They have one goal: *sell stuff!* Their marketing professionals craft meaningless taglines on their products like "#1 pediatrician recommended!" Those labels mean zilch. Even those of us who are trying to shop natural and clean might be washing our kids' hands with toxic chemicals. My clients say, "But, Tonya, I shop at health food stores. They check to make sure everything is safe, right?" Wrong.

If you feel duped, you're not alone. First, let's clear up what I mean by the word *chemical*. Just as there are naturally occurring toxins in our environment, there are also naturally occurring chemicals. In fact, just about everything is a chemical! A chemical is any substance that consists of matter. So that essentially means anything that you can touch—a liquid, a solid, or a gas. So in our natural environment, there are naturally occurring chemicals all around us—the oxygen we breathe, the water we drink, and the granite rocks we climb on when we go hiking. And even naturally occurring chemicals can be toxic. Ever heard of Botox? Of course you have. But did you know that its source is naturally occurring botulinum, one of the deadliest substances known to man? Just one gram of botulinum, which is produced by the bacterium *Clostridium botulinum*, could kill about one million people if it spread. The point here is that natural *and* artificial chemicals can cause harm or hurt. The substance isn't what determines toxicity but rather the dose. Even water can poison us if we drink too much of it.

While you might think chemical-laden products are relatively new, they've actually been around for ages. Human beings have been creating things with chemicals since about 1000 BC. By that time in our history, our forebears were fermenting beer and wine as well as extracting chemicals from plants to make medicines, soaps, and perfumes. What *is* new is the recent explosion of chemical production. In the last fifty years, the production of artificially made chemicals in the United States has skyrocketed.[2] At the same time, there's been a marked increase in the incidence of conditions like attention deficit hyperactivity disorder (ADHD), autism, childhood cancers, diabetes, and obesity.[3] This isn't to say that the rise in artificially made chemicals is the sole catalyst for problems in children's health, but it's interesting to note the correlation. Correlation isn't causation, of course, but as you will learn in this book, science does link certain chemicals to particular health problems.

Today, there are well over forty thousand man-made chemical substances registered on the Toxic Substances Control Act (TSCA) Inventory.[4] While the TSCA is a law created to regulate harmful substances, it's been highly ineffective. Most of those registered substances—around 98 percent—have never been tested for safety by the Environmental Protection Agency (EPA). So in terms of artificial chemicals, it's like the Wild West out there. The onus is on us as consumers to ensure that what we're eating, breathing, and putting in our bodies is safe. Scientists have only begun to scratch the surface of understanding the long-term impact of chemical exposure. This brings me back to my *no guilt* rule. Even scientists and professionals working at the EPA don't know everything about how chemical exposure impacts health. But the health threat from synthetic chemicals is real and backed by mounting scientific evidence.

The influx of chemicals in our lives is compounded by an epidemic of misinformation. Most online information about toxicity in everyday products is dead wrong. According to a study conducted by the Credibility Coalition and published by *Fast Company*, 75 percent of the top ten most-shared health articles in 2018 "contained false or misleading information and exaggerated potential dangers," according to scientists.[5]

For example, I see statements like this all the time: "Twenty-six seconds is all it takes for the chemicals in personal care products to enter your bloodstream."

But that's not necessarily true! First, not all chemicals pass through the skin. For those that do, the speed at which they are absorbed and enter your bloodstream depends on a wide range of different factors, like the concentration of chemicals, where direct skin contact occurs, and how long the contact lasts. It also depends on things like the temperature of your skin and whether or not your skin is damaged.[6]

The bottom line is that it's hard to separate toxin facts from fiction. Even when an online article is backed by "research," you need to dig deeper. Companies that manufacture toxic products will often fund biased studies to "prove" they are safe. But when was the last time you read a health article and then thought, *Better make sure that study was peer reviewed?*

Companies that manufacture products with synthetic chemicals often claim their products are "safe" because they use trace amounts, and in some cases, a much higher dose was deemed safe in animal testing. But little is understood about the synergistic effects of synthetic chemicals—in other words, how they interact with one another in the moment as well as over time. According to researchers at the Institute of Environmental Medicine, it's long been known that there can be synergistic, toxic effects of supposedly safe synthetic chemicals when combined or mixed, but the full extent is often unclear.[7] There simply isn't much research on this topic, as chemical interactions in the human body are challenging to measure and monitor.

Why should you trust me?

You might be wondering why, if there's so much misinformation about environmental toxins, my advice is worth trusting. How do you know that what I say is true? To start, every piece of advice I give in this book is backed by my educational training and research. In 2019, I was named environmental toxin expert of the year by the International Association of Top Professionals. I have a decade of professional experience in holistic nutrition and almost two decades of experience educating the public on products and toxins that affect their health and well-being. And the most important reason I always like to point out: I'm a mom who had to help her child. When people reach out to me for help, it's usually for one of two reasons: they're experiencing a health issue (like allergies, skin irritation, or attention issues), or they know they need to eliminate toxins in their home but don't know how. Most clients have no idea how "safe" chemicals in their homes can interact to disrupt just about every single function in the body. How could they? In this book, I'll share the highlights you need to know that will help you get started right away on creating a healthier home for you and your family.

When I first realized the full scope of harm hiding in everyday products, I was ready to quit. *Fine, toxins, you win.* If you're feeling furious that you've been consuming nasty chemicals and loading your cabinets with a plethora of toxins, take a deep breath. I did too. Every client I've ever worked with did the same thing. It's easy to wonder: *If everything is bad for us, why bother?*

If you're reading this book, my suspicion is that you *do* want to bother—at least some of the time—for the sake of your health and that of the people you love. If you use safe products most of the time, you don't have to worry about what's in everything *all* the time. You don't have to toss out *everything*. It's OK to be mad though. Let's indulge in a primal scream together: *Uggggh!*

Feel better? I do.

Now, let's take back control.

My story

I grew up in the 1980s in Big Rock, Illinois. In our little town just outside Chicago, everyone knew one another. My childhood there was normal and happy. I climbed trees, went for hikes in the woods, and ran next door to play at my grandparents' house. Then, two weeks before my seventh birthday, everything changed. I felt a terrible pain in my back and couldn't raise my arm past shoulder height. When I collapsed while trying to pick up our cat, my parents called the pediatrician. Within minutes, we were racing to his office.

"There's no time to pack," he said. "You need to get to the hospital now." Once there, the doctors ran a battery of tests. My parents wondered if I'd even survive the weekend. Soon, my test results came in. It was a worst-case scenario. I was diagnosed with acute lymphocytic leukemia. At the time, the survival rate was 20 percent. For the next three years, I endured chemotherapy, a slew of painful tests—like bone marrow aspirations, spinal taps, and biopsies—as well as experimental treatments and hospitalizations. I also learned I might not be able to have kids. In fourth grade, I finished chemotherapy, and by middle school, I was playing sports and starting to go back to a pretty normal childhood.

An important lesson from that time stuck with me: a healthy diet and environment are immensely powerful. My oncologist at that time told me to eat nutritious foods, like fruits and vegetables, and to avoid processed food. I learned at a young age that hot dogs, chips, and cookies are bad for your health.

When my kids were born, thankfully proving my oncologist's prediction about my fertility wrong, I paid close attention to their diet. I chose the healthiest foods and the safest products—or so I thought.

In 2006, when my son Eric was eight years old, his second-grade teacher called me and suggested testing him for ADHD. It was tough news, but I wasn't entirely surprised. I'd noticed the symptoms. He tapped his pen incessantly on his desk. He stared out the window and struggled to follow directions with more than two steps.

I thought back to the advice my childhood oncologist gave me and wondered, *Could there be something in our home aggravating Eric's symptoms?* I wanted more time to investigate before pursuing tests. I asked Eric's teacher for more time, and she agreed.

Then I went berserk.

I spent hours on Google looking for things that could have caused his symptoms. Eventually, I discovered that preservatives (such as sodium benzoate) and artificial colors could contribute to the "brain fog" he was experiencing at school.[8] My heart sank; I felt like it was my fault. Even worse, I didn't know what to do about it. After more research, I learned that every "natural" product I had in my pantry was full of preservatives, artificial colors, and fake flavors. I felt ashamed and guilty, and I quickly tossed out everything with those ingredients.

Soon after making some changes in his diet, there was a noticeable effect in Eric's behavior. Just a few weeks later, he was better able to focus. He woke up with more energy and could pay attention to anything—TV, homework, and lessons in school—for longer periods of time. He didn't fidget as much or get out of his chair as often. Just a few small changes to his environment made a tremendous impact on his life. The next month, I sat down with his teacher again.

"His attention has significantly improved," she said. "I don't see a need to test him for ADHD anymore."

I was ecstatic and relieved.

Then I had an idea. *If Eric's attention issues improved after just a few weeks, imagine the profound impact of small changes over a lifetime.*

We didn't "cure" Eric. He was (and still is) an easily distracted kid. We love him exactly the way he is, and he's the first to laugh about those absentmindedness moments. Diet changes alone won't necessarily make a difference for every child experiencing these kinds of symptoms, nor are they a cure-all. However, I was floored by the results I saw with my son. I'm not at all suggesting that my methods are a magic bullet to eliminate ADHD or other cognitive issues. You should always consult with your doctor and never go off medication that a physician has recommended without their input. Instead, I see these strategies as a bonus, an important—and sometimes missing—piece of the puzzle in overall health.

After Eric's attention issues improved, I continued my research. I knew there were other families in the same position—and I wanted to help them. I went back to school and got a master's degree and a board certification in holistic nutrition. Driven by the idea that small changes can go a long way, I created a business to help families have a slightly greener but significantly healthier lifestyle while still enjoying frozen pizza and bright red lipstick.

Now that I'm an environmental health expert, I'm frequently asked to speak on TV shows and the radio. And over time, I realized that after all the hours of research and study, I had become an expert. But most important of all, I'm a mom on a mission.

The pitfalls of going too far

Before I developed the methods in this book, I made an ill-fated attempt at being *aggressively* greener. It didn't work. And it drove my whole family slightly insane.

Initially, I started out with small changes to Eric's diet. But soon, I got carried away. As I researched and learned more about hidden toxins, I accelerated from *a few* small changes to *a lot* of them.

"Are we *ever* going to eat hot dogs again?"

My four-year-old daughter, Lyndsey, said this to me one night. She blinked up at me over a plate of brussels sprouts, that night's dinner. Her normally sparkling blue eyes looked sad. Lyndsey *loves* hot dogs. But after I learned they contain nitrates, which are linked to childhood leukemia, I wouldn't let her eat a single one.[9]

Picture the scene: During the day, I maniacally tossed out everything in our home I suspected of having harmful toxins. I walked around with a giant trash bag, filling it to the brim with forbidden items, bidding adieu to the offending products.

So long, Oreos. I sure did enjoy your creamy filling.

Farewell, delicious potato chips. It was fun while it lasted.

"Popcorn's safe, right?" my husband asked one day, chomping on a few tasty kernels.

"No, it's the worst one!" I snatched the bag of popcorn from his hands and added it to the bulging trash bag. His mouth gaped open.

Next, I went through the bathrooms. Favorite shampoos and deodorants were added to the trash.

At night, while everyone else in my house slept, I Googled information about toxins like a madwoman. The house was dark. I sat on the sofa alone with my worry, staring into the backlight of my laptop. With each click, I grew more paranoid about the dangers lurking in our home. With each study I read, my "things to throw out tomorrow" list grew longer: scented candles, fabric softener, soap. Once I finished Googling for the evening, I'd whip up a batch of DIY sunscreen or a lotion bar. Suddenly, it was three in the morning. I'd crash into bed, my husband beside me, and fall asleep. The next day, I'd wake up bleary eyed and do it all over again.

Would you want to live in this house?

My family certainly didn't. Heck, I didn't either!

I was sleep-deprived, going a wee bit insane, and driving everyone else in my house completely nuts. Oh, and my all-in approach was back-firing. My kids weren't just eating the very processed foods I was working so hard to remove; they were inhaling them like trash compactors every time I wasn't around. I may have eliminated toxic chemicals from our home, but I'd replaced it with a boatload of toxic stress, overwhelming feelings, deprivation, and more than a little resentment.

When Lyndsey looked up at me in the kitchen that night,

crocodile tears welling in the corners of her sweet eyes, it dawned on me. *We've lost some of our joy.* The bliss that comes from biting into a grilled hot dog—that smoky taste, the warm juice dissolving onto your tongue. The fun of getting dressed for a date night with my husband, covering my lashes with a few swipes of mascara, softening my skin with a dollop of scented lotion. The refreshed feeling that comes from getting eight hours of sleep.

I reached a breaking point. And I wondered: *Is this really making us healthier? If so, at what cost?*

I knew there had to be a better way. And that's when I officially became *slightly* greener—this time, for good.

I didn't want my kids growing up saying "I can't have that." Instead, I wanted them to learn how to make better choices on their own. I wanted to teach them how to self-regulate—just like they would need to with screen time, romantic partners, glasses of wine, or anything else in life. When my kids realized how much better they felt once we'd removed the worst chemicals in our home, they started to come around to say, "I don't want to have that." *I can't* means someone else has decided for you; you have no control. *I don't want to* means you've decided for yourself—you're in control. I want everyone—kids, parents, anyone who wants to be healthier—to realize how much control they really have.

We're in this together

If I can follow this lifestyle, anyone can. I seriously can burn a pot of boiling water. (Just ask my kids; it's *that* bad.) I still enjoy making my own cleaners, lotion bars, or toothpaste occasionally. And if I don't have time, I buy a brand I've researched and found to be safer than the conventional alternative, and I'm OK with that. The good news is that there are a lot of safer brands out there. You just need to know what to look for, and that's what this book will help you do.

I'm not going to make you throw out your favorite mascara. You won't have to make your own toilet bowl cleaner. I promise not to push wheatgrass shots. But you can if you want to. That's the beauty of the Slightly Greener Method. You can customize it to fit your lifestyle and needs.

Some people I meet are "power greeners," who go all-in and make eliminating toxins an obsession or a career. The majority of people are either what I call "easy greens" or "over being green." Easy greens are those who implement "easy" green habits (think choosing the "natural" label) with the best of intentions; they *think* these changes are helping them detoxify their environment, even if they aren't. And the "over being green" are those people who have tried, failed, or simply become exhausted, confused, or overwhelmed and decided to quit what feels like a losing battle. It's entirely up to you how green you want to be. If you want to be a power greener—go for it! And if not, that's OK too. I think we all need permission not to be perfect. Whatever your shade of green, we are partners in this lifestyle together. Armed with the tips in the book, we can sleep better, breathe better, feel better. *Live* better.

Because Cheetos taste even more delicious after a day of tossing phthalates in the trash.

2

Getting Started with the Slightly Greener Method

It's easy to let this toxin stuff get the best of you. You can start out with good intentions. *Small changes—I'm in!* But the next thing you know, you're freaking out, convincing your partner to move into a rustic hut, eat leaves, and use mud as body wash. *Whoops, went too far.* In the next section, I'm going to start explaining more about how toxins cause harm and disease in the body. But a warning: this is where fear can creep in.

Before we dig into a little science, repeat after me: "I promise to remember that I don't have to immediately get rid of *every* toxin in my home to be healthy. It's better to be *slightly* greener and stick with it over time."

OK, ready? Let's dive in.

What you need to know about toxins

There are several different ways that toxins can cause harm in the body. (Again, the synthetic chemicals we're discussing are more accurately called *toxicants*, but remember: we're keeping things light here in the *no scare zone*.) The primary toxins found in consumer products and in the environment are carcinogens, mutagens, teratogens, allergens, neurotoxins, and endocrine disruptors. *Carcinogens* are chemicals that cause cancer, like cigarette smoke. *Mutagens* are chemical compounds or forms of radiation (like UV light or X-rays) that can cause mutations in DNA. *Teratogens* are substances, like mercury, that may cause defects in the human embryo. *Allergens* are substances that trigger a response that starts in the immune system and can result in an allergic reaction, like asthma. And then there are *endocrine disruptors*, which are something, usually a man-made chemical, that disrupts or alters the endocrine system, typically by blocking or mimicking hormones, or by causing an over- or underproduction of hormones. I place particular focus on them, because they hide in household products like food, skin care, or over-the-counter medications like acetaminophen or aspirin and wreak havoc all over the body. Substances like phthalates, parabens, and flame retardants can also hide in furniture, dish soap, and makeup. They can mimic hormones, causing health problems like weight gain, insulin resistance, diabetes, allergies, asthma, cardiovascular disease, fertility issues, thyroid problems, an increased cancer risk, and even neurodevelopmental disorders, like ADHD, autism, and lower IQ.[1] In this book, I'll teach you about the most dangerous toxins and how to avoid them with simple changes to the way you shop.

How toxins enter the body and cause harm

If there are toxins in many household products, how exactly do they cause us harm? How do they even get into the body? I used to think that toxins entered the body through one channel—the mouth. You are what you eat, right? From my experience with childhood leukemia, I knew there were things that were "bad for you" in food. But what I didn't know was that toxins can also enter our bodies through the air we breathe as well as the lotions and shampoos we rub on our skin. Toxins are in the cars we drive, the airplanes we fly in, the offices we sit in all day, the schools we send our children to, the furniture we come home to at the end of the day, and the technology we use, in addition to the personal care products we clean ourselves with and the air we breathe outside. The pervasiveness of toxins can contribute to an all (*I must toss everything!*) or nothing (*forget it, can't win!*) approach to managing exposure.

But just as I recommend a little-by-little strategy for making healthy changes, I also recommend the same framework for learning about toxins. It's like learning to swim; if you go straight to the deep end on your first day in the pool, you might drown.

So we'll start by dipping our toes into the waters of environmental toxins, taking one topic at a time.

Endocrine disruptors

Since I focus on endocrine disruptors with many clients, we'll start there. I spend lots of time talking about them for two reasons: first, because they can cause health issues in so many different parts of the body, and second, because they hide in what feels like almost every product we use. Reducing your exposure to endocrine disruptors is a low-effort, high-reward act for your health. They are found in plastic bottles, metal cans, some medicines, flame retardants (which are frequently found in fabrics such as clothes, furniture upholstery, and airline seats), pesticides, children's toys, and cosmetics.[2] They can pose the greatest risk during prenatal and early postnatal development when organs and neural systems are developing.[3] As you might guess from their name, endocrine disruptors cause health problems by interfering with the endocrine system. The endocrine system is comprised of eight different glands that regulate different functions in the body; it's where hormones are made, stored, and secreted. When you see the word *hormones*, you might first think of the reproductive system and puberty. But hormones are responsible for far more than our ability to procreate. In fact, hormones regulate just about every function in the body. Our sleep, appetite, mood, blood sugar, heart rate, thyroid, fertility, blood pressure, and immune system are all managed by hormones. Obviously, none of those functions is one you would want to have disrupted.

When you breathe in flame retardants from the fabric on your sofa, eat canned food that came from a container lined with bisphenol A (BPA), or rub lotion that contains parabens onto your skin, endocrine disruptor chemicals can enter your body. When that happens, your hormones are prevented from effectively doing their job regulating functions like your sleep, mood, or immune response. Endocrine disruptors can produce hormones that aren't needed, cause too many (or too few) hormones to be produced, block existing hormones from doing their job, or imitate certain hormones. In each of these instances, hormone disruption can cause all kinds of health issues. Problems can result in the brain (learning issues, lowered IQ), in the immune system (allergies, autoimmune problems, even cancer), and perhaps most surprising of all, in metabolism regulation and weight.[4]

One particular category of endocrine disruptors that we will cover is called obesogens. *Obesogens* are chemicals that can promote obesity by increasing the number of fat cells or the storage of fat in existing cells. They can even alter how your body metabolizes food or how it recognizes the feeling of being full.[5] But together we will review how you can safely avoid them and keep your kids away from them too. Whew. OK, that is a lot to digest, and we've only covered endocrine disruptors.

Take a deep breath and remember: *small steps.*

Toxins can affect so many different areas of health, even ones you might not expect, like weight, sleep, IQ, and allergies. But in the next few pages, you will learn three easy tips that you can implement right away to avoid many of them.

Carcinogens, allergens, and neurotoxins

While endocrine disruptors are the toxin category we'll examine most carefully throughout this book, you will also learn how to avoid carcinogens, allergens, and neurotoxins. *Carcinogens* are substances that can cause cancer.[6] However, just because they *can* cause cancer does not mean they *will*. Some carcinogens are fairly easy to avoid, like cigarette smoke or the sun's rays. Others are more challenging to escape because they hide in the air we breathe, the food we eat, or the products we use. When you are exposed to a carcinogen, it can cause changes to certain genes in the body, which alter the way some cells function. But there are many factors that influence whether that will happen, including your genetic makeup and how long (or how intensely) you were exposed. In each section of this book, I will teach you how to avoid known carcinogens that can hide in common products.

Allergens are any substance that can cause an immune response, which tends to provoke symptoms like itchy eyes or runny nose. Though you may first think food, pollen, or pet dander as the typical causes of an allergic response, substances in consumer products can be the culprit too. Fragrances, preservatives, dyes, and pesticides can also trigger an allergic reaction or exacerbate allergies.[7]

Neurotoxins are substances in the environment that can negatively impact brain health. They can be found in pesticides or additives in our food, cosmetics, and certain cleaning solvents. Other neurotoxins in the environment include lead, mercury, ethanol, fluoride, and arsenic. They can disrupt or alter the nervous system or brain in a way that kills nerves and can cause behavioral problems, prematurity, and intellectual deficits.

As you will see through the book, some substances can fall into multiple categories of toxins, like pesticides. For example, some pesticides can be a neurotoxin (they can cause issues with brain health) *and* an allergen (they can cause an allergic response). Double the reason to stay away.

Why kids are extra vulnerable

No matter the type of toxin, kids (and especially babies) are extra vulnerable. Making small changes to be slightly greener is like snapping them into a car seat, a seat belt for their future health. Children are much more sensitive than adults to toxic chemicals in the environment, and their exposure to the toxins in the air, in food, and in water are far greater.[8] Because of their low body weight, children are exposed to a higher potency of toxins than adults. Kids take in an average of three to four more calories per pound than adults, and a six-month-old infant consumes seven times more water per pound than an adult does.[9] Infants also take in twice as much air per pound as adults do. These differences mean that kids are disproportionately exposed to harmful chemicals in food, water, and air. This is further amplified by the fact that kids touch everything and then put their hands in their mouths.

Children also have immature metabolic pathways, meaning they have a less developed detoxification system in the body. They haven't yet developed the enzymes to break down and flush toxic chemicals out of the body. For all these reasons, kids are more at risk to the harmful effects of environmental toxins. Very young children face what's called a "window of vulnerability." This is a critical period in early development, between conception and early childhood, where even a very small dose of toxic chemicals can cause problems with organ development or lifelong impairments.[10] Scientists now know that some diseases, like cancer and neurodegenerative diseases, can be caused by processes that may start with exposure in infancy.[11] Kids' extreme vulnerability to environmental toxins is reason enough for significant concern. And since more and more synthetic chemicals are being produced (and few tested for safety) every year, protecting children from harmful chemicals in their environment just seems like a no-brainer.

The good news is that you're already on your way to knowing how to protect your family. The bad news is that babies are exposed to a ton of different chemicals starting in the womb. Children are most susceptible to toxin damage from the time they are in utero until the first few years of life. In 2004, the Environmental Working Group found an average of 287 different industrial chemicals and pollutants in umbilical cord blood of the newborns tested.[12] Among the harmful chemicals found were pesticides, consumer product ingredients, and wastes from burning coal, gasoline, and garbage. Of the 287 different chemicals that were found, 180 are known to cause cancer in humans or animals, 217 are toxic to the brain and nervous system, and 208 cause birth defects or abnormal development in animal studies. One group of chemicals found in this study was perfluorochemicals, which are used in fast-food packaging and water- and stain-resistant clothing. One specific perfluorochemical the researchers found was the Teflon chemical perfluorooctanoic acid, which has recently been characterized as a likely human carcinogen by the EPA's Science Advisory Board.[13] The study also found brominated flame retardants and numerous pesticides too. In short, children today are exposed to *a lot* of different chemicals that are known to cause serious harm. It shouldn't be this way. Kids should live in a world in which they can be born free of harmful toxin exposure. But there are simple ways to reduce this exposure.

The health challenges facing children extend far beyond infancy. It's concerning to consider what might be causing them. Today, one in five children has a diagnosed learning disorder.[14] Childhood obesity rates in the United States have tripled among two- to nineteen-year-olds since 1980.[15] Children born in the U.S. have a 34.5 percent chance of developing asthma, allergies, eczema, or hay fever.[16] Rates of invasive pediatric cancers are up over 20 percent in the last twenty years, and a study released by the CDC in 2013 revealed that food allergies in children increased by approximately 50 percent between 1997 and 2011.[17] Those are some pretty staggering statistics. While harmful chemical exposure is likely not to blame for every one of these health issues, there are plenty of instances in which there is a known connection between a chemical commonly found in our everyday lives and health problems. And then there are the undiscovered harmful effects of everyday chemicals that we don't know about yet. Think back to the "silent epidemic" of lead poisoning in the 1970s—millions of American children were unnecessarily exposed to lead in gasoline, paint, and even some consumer products. Who knows what chemicals we think are safe today will be deemed unsafe in the future?

If you feel a panicky feeling rising up inside right now, remember: you don't have to (and couldn't possibly) protect your child from every potential toxin. As much as our kids need protection from environmental toxins, they also need parents who are sane, joyful, and balanced. So don't let yourself go cuckoo over this stuff. Take it from me—it doesn't work. You'll crash and burn surrounded by a sea of empty Twinkie wrappers.

But I promise, there's a way to achieve balance.

Define your why

When I first meet with a client, my job is to teach them to set up systems to eliminate my job. Sounds crazy, but that's the truth! My process includes helping clients figure out *which* small changes they need to make and how they can build on them over time. So before we go into detail on the holistic lifestyle tips I recommend, we'll start by having you *define your why*.

First, take a little time and write down why you bought this book. Stumped? Here are a few questions I ask clients:

▸ What's prompting your desire to be greener?

▸ Are you concerned with overall toxicity?

▸ Did you hear about obesogens and think maybe that's why you can't lose weight?

▸ Are you worried about a sick family member who is just not getting better?

▸ Are you (or is someone in your home) having health issues in any of the following areas?

Circle all that apply for you:

- ▸ Allergies
- ▸ Asthma
- ▸ Attention issues
- ▸ Autoimmune disorder
- ▸ Behavior issues
- ▸ Diabetes
- ▸ Eczema
- ▸ Headaches
- ▸ Learning disabilities
- ▸ Mood issues
- ▸ Thyroid issues/weight gain

Or maybe you don't have any health issues but just want to live a healthier lifestyle? That's great!

Eric's second-grade teacher provided my wake-up call, and whenever my teenage daughters give me the side-eye about not eating processed snack foods or my husband brings home a toxic cleaning product instead of the safer brand I asked him to buy—*again*—I remember why I decided to live by the Slightly Greener Method in the first place. My why is to ensure that my family stays healthy without losing our sanity or hot dogs.

Your why might be totally different from mine—or anyone else's—and that's OK. Some of my clients' whys have included wanting to solve a specific health challenge (like skin or breathing issues) or a desire to lose weight or feel healthier. Some people want to reduce stress; they have nagging anxiety that they keep unsafe products in their homes but don't know where to start to create change. Some want to create an environment safe for kids. Once you know your why, it will help you figure out exactly where to begin your slightly greener approach. It will also be what keeps you committed going forward, when those small changes (at first!) feel invisible. Sometimes, it takes sticking with the changes for a little while to see or feel the difference. So when you're tempted to just throw in the towel, you'll remember why you decided to follow the Slightly Greener Method in the first place.

Knowing your why is also important for explaining the changes to everyone you live with. When you explain the why behind your actions to your child, they tend to make good decisions themselves too. For example, Eric was a wrestler as a child, and at that time, he also had issues with asthma. Like most kids, he loved Popsicles. My husband liked to buy the brightly colored ones filled with food coloring. One day—to my horror—I found Eric eating a yellow Popsicle. But instead of slapping it out of his hand like I wanted to, I took a gentler route. I explained to him that FD&C Yellow No. 5, the dye that provided the sunshine-yellow color, was linked to worsening asthma symptoms.[18] I went on to explain that eating food like that Popsicle might negatively affect his physical fitness and wrestling performance. He took one look at the Popsicle and then threw it away. #MomWin.

Knowing your why will also help you focus on which changes are most important *for you*. If your why means addressing your hair loss, you can focus on personal care products, and you don't need to overhaul your pantry yet. There's no need to feel overwhelmed about all the safer, healthier choices you *could* make. Revisiting your why often will remind you to stay focused on the most important changes and make it easy on yourself. And then you can stay committed!

If you're not struggling with any specific health issues at the moment, I suggest that you focus first on avoiding endocrine disruptors, because they can cause so many different health problems in the body, especially in children. Start there, and implement just a few changes at a time.

Three tips for becoming slightly greener

At its most basic level, the Slightly Greener Method comes down to three easy tips. And if you remember and implement these three things when cleaning your house, shopping for groceries, and buying personal care products, you'll already be slightly greener.

Tip #1: Memorize your deal breakers

Single people often have deal breakers while dating (you know, like when you find out you're dating the guy who claps when the plane lands); now you'll have them for products you bring into your home. Once you establish deal breakers, you'll be able to tell right away whether a product is acceptable. For example, because we have ADHD and learning disabilities in my family, my deal breaker ingredients include monosodium glutamate (MSG), artificial colors, and benzoate preservatives. All these ingredients have been shown to negatively affect learning and cognition.[19] When I go grocery shopping,

I check the ingredient labels on every single product. If I see any of those ingredients, I put the package back on the shelf. After practicing this habit for a while, it becomes automatic—I know which products are safe and what to avoid.

Tip #2: The 80/20 rule

The 80/20 rule works for so many things in life, doesn't it? If you can buy safer products 80 percent of the time, then you don't have to worry so much over the 20 percent of the time you can't control. Whether it's for budget reasons, or you're traveling and forget an item and the store doesn't carry a safer version, or even just because you want to treat yourself occasionally without guilt, the 80/20 rule comes in handy. If 80/20 seems out of reach, that's fine too. Start with 40/60, 50/50, or whatever works for you, your budget, and your lifestyle.

Tip #3: Find your top two

Another simple way to make your home slightly greener is to identify one or two of the most-used, most-consumed products in each category—eating, skin and body, and cleaning—and replace those first. For example, my daughter loves hot dogs, but I try to avoid them. Studies have shown that they contain nitrites, nitrates, and nitrosamines, which are linked to childhood cancer and leukemia.[20] So for me, it was easy to select hot dogs as one food product to eliminate. But since we are going *slightly* greener here—with an eye for the long term and sustainability—I didn't rule them out completely. So as a treat, I do buy hot dogs every once in a while. But I always purchase a safer brand, Applegate Farms, because their hot dogs do not contain GMOs, antibiotics, or artificial ingredients like sodium nitrate (a chemical also found in fireworks) or sodium diacetate (an ingredient in chemical hand warmers). This way, my daughter still gets the occasional treat, and I feel better about what's *in* the hot dog she's eating.

The bottom line

If you apply these three tips, you may start to see positive changes quickly. I know I did. My method is reasonable, simple, and doable. You don't need to memorize a bunch of weird scientific ingredients. You won't drive anyone crazy by being slightly greener. But you'll get all the benefits. Remember, you don't need to do every single thing in this book to have a clean, pretty, and—most important—healthy home.

3

The Power of
Starting Small

My client Sarah from Indiana came to me when her hair started falling out. She was desperate for a solution to her hair loss. But she was also skeptical that a small change—like switching to a different shampoo brand—could help. While there are certainly other causes for hair loss, I suggested that Sarah try tossing out her old shampoo and replacing it with a sulfate-free brand.

"Really, just a few days with new shampoo might help?" Sarah asked.

"Yes, it might," I told her. "Stick with it and report back."

Most shampoos, as well as many other products like toothpaste and dish soap, contain sodium lauryl sulfate (SLS). SLS is the ingredient that creates that satisfying lather in your hair and on your hands when you wash your hair or clean dishes, but it's not necessary for cleaning purposes. We've been conditioned to believe that the *suds* are what does the cleaning, but they are just a chemical byproduct. SLS can cause skin and gum irritation, hair breakage, even hair loss. Exactly the opposite of what you want from your shampoo!

When I explained this to Sarah, she breathed a sigh of relief knowing that she didn't have to turn her entire life upside down to address her hair problem. Sure enough, a few days after switching brands of shampoo, she noticed less hair falling out. Eventually, it significantly improved. Energized by her initial success, Sarah switched to a different brand of body lotion too. Then came changes to her toothpaste and skin care products, until the majority of her self-care products were free of the most harmful chemicals. I see clients experience transformations like Sarah's all the time. People are shocked to learn how effective small changes can be.

Time and time again, I've found that my clients were paralyzed by the persistent cultural myth that "detoxifying" your home means getting rid of every single harmful product. This couldn't be further from the truth. Scientific research reveals that reducing your overall exposure to harmful chemicals impacts your long-term health.[1] Increasingly, studies are showing that changes to your diet and the products you use, even just in the short term, lower the toxin buildup in your body.[2] One study showed that after just one week of eating organic produce, pesticide levels in participants' urine dropped by almost 60 percent![3] I've seen these dramatic results after small changes in my clients too.

Toni in South Carolina had a three-year-old daughter with sleep issues and allergies. Together, we deduced that some harmful ingredients in her daughter's diet—such as artificial colors and BHT, which is a preservative used to keep packaged foods fresh—might be the cause. Sure enough, after a few small dietary changes as well as removing artificial fragrances in her home, Toni's daughter started sleeping better and had fewer stuffy noses. It's hard for people to see that tiny little changes matter to your health, but they do.

Long-term exposure to chemicals over decades has a significant impact on health. A growing body of evidence suggests that our exposure to these chemicals is contributing to a wide range of chronic diseases and illnesses.[4] One study found that just *three days* of eliminating endocrine disruptors from personal care products reduced overall exposure by an average of 35 percent.[5] By reducing their exposure, not only did my clients Sarah and Toni improve their hair, skin, allergy, and sleep issues, but it's entirely possible that they also prevented future illnesses, like cancer, autoimmune conditions, or thyroid issues.

As exposure to toxic chemicals has expanded dramatically over the past century, the number of people exposed has ballooned, even if they are only experiencing lower levels of exposure. But researchers are now realizing that it's not just big exposures that cause illness. In fact, the number of people who have low to moderate exposures to toxins and will ultimately develop a disease is significantly larger than the number of people who get a disease from being heavily exposed.[6] People have varying degrees of sensitivity to harmful toxins and respond to chemical exposures in different ways. Some people might experience exposure and never get sick, while others might be more sensitive and get sick from that same level of exposure.[7] Some diseases are caused by chemical exposures (like learning disabilities caused by lead exposure), while other diseases (like asthma) are exacerbated by them. We don't yet fully understand why some people are more susceptible to becoming ill from toxins. However, we do know that it isn't realistic or necessary to reduce toxin exposure to zero. As consumers, this is great news, because it means we need to make wise choices overall, but we don't have to be perfect every single day.

How the body filters toxins

The human body is quite skilled at regulating itself and filters most toxins on its own. The body's liver, kidneys, and lymphatic system are designed to remove harmful substances.[8] When the body takes in a toxin (either through food, air, medication, or absorption by the skin), that toxin is then metabolized by enzymes primarily located in the liver.[9] The toxins are essentially broken down by the enzymes so that they can be eliminated from the body through feces, urine, or sweat. The effectiveness of those enzymes depends on a number of factors, including genetics, diet, environmental toxins, medication, and nutritional status.[10]

When these detoxification systems become overwhelmed, toxin overload occurs—the body is taking in more toxins than it can deal with. The human body is a complex ecosystem, and when illness occurs, it's because the body's homeostasis has been disrupted in some way.[11] Every biological regulating system in the body has a threshold, a tipping point. The body can only handle so much, and when the enzyme pathways become overloaded with an excess of toxins, it will then become dysregulated and fail.[12] And that is when illness can set in.

This is why the Slightly Greener Method is effective. The goal is to avoid toxic overload by reducing your overall exposure long-term.

How toxins build up in the body

Body burden (also called toxic load) is the concentration or amount of a chemical in the body at any given time.[13] Some chemicals (like certain pesticides) are what's called *water soluble*, meaning they can dissolve in water and leave the body fairly quickly, through our urine or feces.[14] But some chemicals, such as mercury, don't dissolve in water and are instead stored in fat and are not as easily removed from the body. Chemicals also have what's called a *biological half-life*, which is the time that it takes to reduce the concentration in the body by one-half. Some toxins have a longer half-life and simply take much longer to exit the body.[15] Repeat exposure (like repeatedly spritzing that same air freshener in your home) will also result in cumulative buildup (known as bioaccumulation) and increase body burden.[16] You can see bioaccumulation in people who work in nail salons or other jobs where they are exposed to harmful chemicals each day. Each one of us has *some* level of industrial chemical buildup in our bodies, as evidenced by residues that can be found in human blood, urine, or breast milk. The goal is to keep that buildup as low as possible.

There are a variety of factors that influence chemical storage in the body, including the dosage (how much you were exposed to), duration of exposure, how much time passed in between exposures, interaction with other chemicals, age, sex, and your general health. If you generally practice healthy lifestyle behaviors, this will help! Regular exercise, a healthy diet, stress reduction, and not smoking will all boost your body's ability to effectively eliminate toxins.

Children's detoxification systems aren't sophisticated enough to take on extra chemicals and flush them out of the body quickly, so it's especially important to eliminate unnecessary toxins from their environment whenever possible.[17] Toxic overload can take a significant toll on your child's health and can negatively affect academic performance and behavior too. In some instances, chemicals are known to specific illnesses; in some cases, that link is certain (like known carcinogens, which are known to cause cancer), and in others, there is a suspected but uncertain link. The synergistic effects have not been studied, as they are challenging to measure and trace.[18] How can you possibly measure the interaction of dryer sheet fragrance and sunscreen spray absorbed in combination into your body?

The READ method

When I work with my clients, many of them want a quick takeaway they can implement right off the bat to make their home healthier. To meet that need, I developed the READ method, which provides four simple steps you can remember for creating a healthier home right away. The READ method will not only have a big impact, but it only requires a small amount of effort to get started.

R = *Replace plastic around foods and beverages*

E = *Eat organic and whole foods*

A = *Avoid artificial fragrance*

D = *Destroy dust*

Following all four steps is great, but if you can't, start by doing one or two as often as you can, and then add another step once you get one or two under your belt. Remember, the focus is on *progress* and *balance*. We'll go through each basic READ step in the next few pages and then explore these topics much deeper later in the book.

R = Replace plastic around your foods and beverages

The *R* is for replacing plastic food containers and water bottles, as these can contain chemicals such as BPA (bisphenol A, an endocrine disruptor) and phthalates (another endocrine disruptor) that can leach into foods and beverages. These chemicals can disrupt hormones by affecting the endocrine system, which we now know regulates every function of the body. BPA and phthalates have also been linked to lower IQ and behavior issues in children.[19] Chemicals can leach into foods and beverages when the container or reusable water bottle is exposed to heat or extreme cold, either through washing in the dishwasher, microwaving, leaving the item in a hot car, placing a hot food or beverage in it, or storing it in the freezer.[20] The first thing to do is to go through your kitchen and replace plastic containers and bottles with glass and stainless-steel options. It can be expensive to do this all at once, so start by going through your cabinets and grabbing all your plastic containers (including items that are labeled BPA-free) and putting them on the counter. Then choose your one or two most-used containers and bottles and replace just those first. Don't replace them with plastic-type products that are labeled as BPA-free, as BPA is typically just substituted with similar chemicals.

Next, make sure you don't expose any plastic that comes into contact with food or beverages to heat or freezing temperatures. This means if you *are* using plastic food containers or plastic baggies, keep them at room temperature and use them for dry foods that are kept at room temperature, like pretzels or trail mix. Make sure not to put plastic in the dishwasher or the microwave, and avoid placing hot foods in plastic containers. Remove the plastic when drinking hot liquids too, such as when you get takeout coffee in a cup with a plastic lid. Washing plastic containers in the sink with soap and warm water is fine, because that water is much cooler than the dishwasher, which heats up to 120°F or higher. Freezing can also cause leaching by breaking down the plastic chemicals, so I recommend you use mason jars, silicone freezer bags, or Pyrex (or another glass food storage option) for freezing food.

Once you've removed your most-used plastic food storage from your kitchen, you will need to replace it with something else. I recommend Lifefactory products for glass water bottle and food storage containers and Klean Kanteen for stainless steel options. S'well also makes stainless steel water bottle options in fun designs! Pyrex is a great option for food storage, and retailers often offer their products on sale, so be sure to check often. And then just replace the rest of your plastic items as needed. Super simple!

E = Eat organic and whole foods

We'll dig into the benefits of organic eating as well as the complexities of the organic industry in much more detail in Chapter 4. But at a high level, organic foods are those produced without using chemically formulated fertilizers, growth stimulants, antibiotics, or pesticides. It's important to know that some pesticides (found on nonorganic produce) are linked to ADHD in children.[21] Some pesticides can act as endocrine disruptors. Perhaps even more appalling, one study calculated a cumulative loss of 16.9 million IQ points in American children due to the use of organophosphate pesticides, which are the most commonly used pesticides in agriculture.[22] So I always recommend that clients eat organic foods as much as possible. Whole foods are plant foods that are unprocessed and unrefined (or minimally processed and refined) before being consumed.[23] These are foods like fruits, vegetables, whole grains, and legumes. As you will learn in the next section, food processing can introduce harmful ingredients into food products. One of the easiest ways to prevent toxin overload is just to avoid them in the first place!

A = Avoid artificial fragrance

You will see fragrance listed as an ingredient on many cosmetic products. It's in personal care products like shampoos, hair spray, body lotions, deodorants, baby wash, baby shampoo, and baby wipes. You will also find it in cleaning products as well as in scented candles and air fresheners. But those lemon, lavender, or rose-smelling scents are often derived from artificial chemicals. In fact, artificial fragrance can be made up of multiple ingredients but is considered to be a "trade secret," so its individual ingredients are not required to be listed on the label. Many of these ingredients are toxic (like carcinogens, allergens, respiratory irritants, and chemicals that are toxic to the brain and nervous system).[24] Plug-in air fresheners let off a constant stream of fragrance, and aerosol spray air fresheners are linked to headaches, depression in adults, and ear infections in infants.[25] Many candles use paraffin wax, which can release toxic fumes such as benzene (a known cancer causer) and styrene and toluene (which can affect the nervous system) when burned.[26]

D = Destroy dust

Ever wondered what's in household dust? At first glance, it looks kind of gross but harmless. But it turns out that dust is essentially a repository for the potpourri of harmful toxins throughout our homes. Teeny littles specks of chemicals that escape from clothing, furniture, cleaning supplies, consumer products, and dirt that we track in on our shoes merge with things like skin flakes, pet dander, and pollen to create dust. Researchers at George Washington University found several harmful chemicals in common household dust, including ones linked to hormone disruption, lower IQ, behavior issues in children, thyroid issues, weight gain, and cancer.[27] The study also found that household dust frequently contains phthalates (which are linked to developmental issues, hormone disruption, reproduction issues, and lower IQ), flame retardants (linked to hormone disruption, behavior and attention issues, and obesity, among other issues), fluorinated chemicals (linked to increased breast cancer risk and altered immune system), and lead (linked to neurological problems and lower IQ).[28] That's a whole lot of different chemicals hiding in your dust! But you don't need to eliminate every speck of dust in your home. Here's a quick dusting tip to get the most out of your efforts: pick one or two rooms where you or your kids spend the most time. Start there, and dust that area one extra time per week. That's it!

One step at a time

In the next three parts of the book, we will break down each category (food, personal care, and cleaning) into much more detail. But before we go on, I want to reiterate how important it is not to take on too much, too fast. There's no judgment on this path, and the most important component of it is that you *stick with it*. Instead of trying everything you learned all at once, pick one or two strategies, and make sure you're staying on track before you add additional steps.

Part II

Slightly Greener Eating

4

Learn to Read Ingredients, Not Labels

"You are what you eat."

This familiar adage was popularized by Victor Lindlahr, a nutritionist and health food writer, who published a book in 1940 with the same name. An early pioneer in the "clean eating" movement, Lindlahr believed that food was a catalyst for good health. Back then, there were only about three thousand different food items available for sale in the average grocery store.[1] Today, that number has swelled to over fifty thousand.[2]

While many of us *want* to do what Lindlahr suggested—eat healthy food—it can be difficult to discern which foods are best.

Our food system is a vast global supply chain stretching from one edge of the earth to the other. Food passes through many hands before it lands in our grocery carts, and at times, it can be hard to know *what* exactly we are eating (or what's been sprayed on or added to it). Even those of us trying to make informed choices can find ourselves fooled by misleading food labels.

I always advise that clients start by taking a close look at what's in their refrigerators, their pantries, and their grocery carts.

"Food is the foundation," I tell them. "Let's start there."

Every single client I've ever had is shocked to learn how they've been misled by the food industry. Many of them were spending dollar after hard-earned dollar on food they *thought* was healthy and safe but often wasn't.

Before they come to me, many clients have fallen prey to what I call the *packaging pitfall*. Images and words on food packages are carefully designed to convey a false sense of safety and health. Most consumers don't realize that the details—the ingredients in the food—are the elements that tell the full story. Rather than trusting what the front of the food package tells you (Natural! Healthy!) you need to learn to examine the list of ingredients on the back. (Is there MSG? Preservatives?) In this section, I will teach you exactly how to read ingredient labels and which ones to look for. If you're thinking, *Tonya, I barely have time to buy the food, much less study it with a microscope!* rest assured. Once you learn the tricks and tips, grocery shopping is simple. You won't have to collect four hundred folders' worth of research just to open a box of crackers.

But before we dive into the specifics of what to look for when you're shopping for food, I want to provide some context behind why it's hard to distinguish food products that *are* safe from the ones simply designed to *look* that way.

We'll start by talking about the term *organic*. Many consumers tend to look at an organic label and think, *I know this means the food is better, healthier* somehow, and plop it in their shopping cart. But what does that term really mean? First, let's take a step back to understand how organic food as we know it came to be.

The history of the organic food movement

J. I. Rodale, the founder of the publishing company Rodale, Inc., is widely known as the founder of the modern organic farming movement.[3] Rodale played a significant role in the development of nonchemical farming methods and drew many of his ideas from a British scientist named Albert Howard. Howard had spent years studying agricultural traditional systems in India, and he was the first Westerner to document the Vedic Indian techniques of sustainable agriculture, which we know today as organic farming.[4] Inspired by Howard's findings, in the early 1940s, Rodale created the magazine *Organic Farming and Gardening* as a vehicle for communicating Howard's ideas, which spawned the first generation of organic farmers in the United States. Rodale advocated partnering with the plant, soil, and animal world to grow food in ecological balance rather than using synthetic fertilizers, pesticides, or other ways of dominating the natural world.

In the 1970s, Rodale's methods gained popularity, fueled by increasing environmental awareness and consumer demand to eliminate pesticide-laden crops and antibiotic-fed livestock and instead protect biodiversity and the health of our ecosystems. But the movement was decentralized and faced challenges since each state had their own standards and regulations, and there wasn't standard, unified oversight. In 1990, the United States Department of Agriculture (USDA) passed the Organic Foods Production Act to establish a national standard for organic food and fiber production. Since then, the organic food market has been growing steadily. However, it still makes up only a tiny fraction of produce grown on farmland in the United States—less than one percent![5] Today, the production techniques used in organic farming are quite similar to the national standards established in 1990.

ORGANIC

This term is highly regulated for food, but it is not regulated for some nonfood products. Whether a food is organic is *not* determined by where you buy it (like farmers markets or health food stores), and not every "organic" label is created equal.

Understanding organic food labels

Today, the National Organic Standards Board, a federal advisory board made up of fifteen dedicated public volunteers from across the organic community, such as scientists, public interest advocates, and environmentalists, oversees the USDA organic label.[6] USDA certified organic products have strict labeling and production requirements that must be met. The U.S. organic industry is regulated by the National Organic Program, which is part of the USDA's Agricultural Marketing Service.[7]

But did you know there are three different levels of organic, only one of which means truly pesticide-free? It's not quite as simple as looking for the word *organic* and calling it a day. There are a few different terms that you may see on the labels of organic (or partially organic) food products. Becoming USDA certified is a rigorous process where certifying agents, who are accredited by the USDA, inspect each step of the production process (growing, processing, packaging, labeling) to make sure that compliance with organic standards is being met at every single step.[8] Once that process is complete, there are four different categories that can be used to market the product to consumers, depending on the specifics of how that product was produced and processed.[9] The guidelines that must be met include the following:

- Synthetic pesticides, chemical fertilizers, or GMOs cannot be used.
- Organic meat, dairy products, and eggs cannot include growth hormones or antibiotics.
- Year-round grazing access and non-GMO feed are required for livestock.
- The farm cannot have used any of the prohibited substances on its land for three years prior to applying for status.

Getting the USDA Organic seal is quite a rigorous process indeed. But many of my clients, like most consumers, aren't fully aware of what the distinction means. So to clarify, here are the different labels you will see and what they signify.[10]

100% Organic (or USDA Organic)

If you see the USDA Organic seal on a product, it means that a food was produced without the use of synthetic pesticides, GMOs, or artificial fertilizers. Organic meat and dairy products with the seal are from animals that were fed organic, vegetarian feed and were not treated with hormones or antibiotics. To get the USDA seal and 100% Organic label is a challenge. It is difficult to make a product that is absolutely 100 percent organic. This means that there cannot be any cross-contamination with nonorganic ingredients in the plant where it is grown (excluding salt and water, which are considered natural), and special practices must be used to stand by this guarantee. For that reason, most products in this category are single ingredient products. Most raw, unprocessed farm products can be designated 100 percent organic. Similarly, farm products that have no added ingredients—such as grain flours or rolled oats—can also be labeled 100 percent organic.

Organic

When you see the word *organic* on the label, this means that at least 95 percent of the ingredients in that product were grown organically. You will see this often because some products may have a minor ingredient that does not have an organic option available. Up to 5 percent of the ingredients may be nonorganic agricultural products (meaning foods that come from plants or animals) and/or nonagricultural products (meaning allowable substances that are used to enhance food, like baking soda) that are on the National List of Allowed and Prohibited Substances.[11] These ingredients are essential in organic food processing but often difficult to get in organic form, either because the supply is quite limited or because the ingredient—as in the instance of baking soda—cannot be certified organic. Those allowable substances also follow a strict set of guidelines that must be followed.

According to the USDA, the substances on that list must meet the following criteria:[12]

1. The substance cannot be produced from a natural source, and there are no organic substitutes.

2. The substance's manufacture, use, and disposal do not have adverse effects on the environment and are done in a manner compatible with organic handling.

3. The nutritional quality of the food is maintained when the substance is used, and the substance itself or its breakdown products do not have an adverse effect on human health as defined by applicable federal regulations.

4. The substance's primary use is not as a preservative or to recreate or improve flavors, colors, textures, or nutritive value lost during processing, except where the replacement of nutrients is required by law.

5. The substance is listed as generally recognized as safe by the Food and Drug Administration (FDA) when used in accordance with the FDA's good manufacturing practices and contains no residues of heavy metals or other contaminants in excess of tolerances set by the FDA.

6. The substance is essential for the handling of organically produced agricultural products.

Made with organic ingredients

If you see the phrase *made with organic ingredients* on the label, this means the product must contain at least 70 percent certified organic ingredients (not including salt or water). These products may contain up to 30 percent of allowed nonorganic ingredients. All ingredients— including the 30 percent nonorganic ingredient—must be produced without GMOs, and each organic ingredient must be listed individually, such as "contains organic strawberries and blueberries."[13]

Foods products that are made with less than 70 percent organic ingredients can't have any of the labels listed above, and there aren't any restrictions on the other ingredients, but they can list organic ingredients in the ingredients section, like you might see a cookie with the ingredients listed as organic oats, milk, eggs, flour, and organic raisins.

The many kinds of eggs

Have you ever noticed how many different labels there are on eggs? *Cage-free. Free range. No antibiotics. Organic.* It should be easy to determine what you're getting when you purchase a dozen eggs, but the labels can be misleading here too. So what do these different labels on egg cartons mean? The following definitions are from the USDA:[14]

Cage-free

These eggs are produced by hens in a building or enclosed area with unlimited access to food and water. It doesn't specify how much room they are given, only that they don't live in cages.

Free range

Eggs from these hens must that have constant access to the outdoors and unlimited access to food and water during their egg-laying cycle. Mesh netting or fencing may constitute the outdoor area.[15]

Omega-3

This means that these eggs come from a "flock fed a diet enhanced with omega-3 fatty acids."[16] This means that the hens have been fed flax seed, which contains high amounts of omega-3 fatty acids. Omega-3 fatty acids have many health benefits, such as fighting inflammation and reducing risk for heart disease and depression, and most people don't consume enough of them.[17]

Vegetarian

To use this term on an egg carton label, the producer must document that no animal byproducts were used in the feed or water source of the flocks.[18]

USDA Organic

To qualify for the USDA Organic certification, eggs must come from hens that were fed organic diets, from grains that are not genetically modified and that were grown on land free from pesticides and fertilizers for at least three years. The hens also cannot be exposed to antibiotics or other drugs.[19]

No hormones

This term is deceptive, because no hormones are ever used in the production of eggs. Like some other food labels we've examined, this one is included with the intent of making consumers think the eggs are somehow healthier than other brands. However, when you do see it on the label, the USDA states in their labeling guidelines that an asterisk must follow the term *No Hormones* and include the phrase "No hormones are used in the production of shell eggs." The same applies if you see the term *No Steroids* on the label.[20]

Organic or conventional produce?

OK, but what about fruits and vegetables? Are those labels different? If you buy organic produce, you're in good company; a study published in 2017 showed that 82 percent of American families buy organic food regularly.[21] If you're not currently shopping organic and you can afford to do so, you should—it's one of the easiest changes you can make for your family, especially shopping for organic produce. It's easy to figure out what's organic in the produce section. Fruits and veggies should all have a PLU sticker. PLU is an acronym for price lookup, and it is the same number grocery cashiers everywhere have to remember or find in the big binder at the register during checkout. But you don't have to memorize every single number in that giant binder. Instead, all you have to do is memorize two of them.

The first number you need to remember is 9. When the PLU sticker starts with 9, the produce is organic. Easy-peasy, right? "If the sticker starts with nine, it's fine." That's how I always remember it when I go to the store. The second number to remember is 4. When you see the number on a PLU sticker start with a 4, the produce is conventional. The way I remember that one is "four is poor."

ON PLU STICKERS

9 is for organic produce. Say it with me—*Nine is fine.*

4 is for conventional produce—*Four is poor.*

Some clients say they are fine with their conventionally grown produce, meaning food that was grown using chemical intervention to fight pests and weeds.[22] While they realize the produce is exposed to pesticides, they think, *Oh, I'll just wash my strawberries. It's fine.* But according to the Environmental Working Group (EWG) 2020 Shopper's Guide to Pesticide in Produce, 70 percent of fresh produce in the United States has pesticide residues on it even after it is washed.[23] The CDC says that a variety of acute as well as chronic health issues are associated with exposures to pesticides. Some affect the nervous system, others may cause cancer or interfere with the endocrine system, while others may irritate the skin or eyes. The CDC says that health risks increase according to the intensity and duration of exposure and points out children are at particular risk.[24] Scientists say it's hard to determine the precise exposure humans have to pesticides in their daily lives and even harder still to determine what their cumulative or synergistic effect might be. According to a 2018 study, 90 percent of Americans have detectable pesticide levels in their urine and blood.[25] Pesticide exposure can cause long-term health problems

like cancer; brain or nervous system damage; birth defects; reproductive problems; or damage to the liver, kidneys, lungs, and other
organs.[26] While there are a variety of ways pesticides can enter the
human body (breathing them in, for example, or absorption through
eyes and skin), the primary route is through diet. The EPA does have
rules for how pesticides are used, but none of the current rules and
restrictions can prevent cumulative exposure over a lifetime.

One particular pesticide that has been in the news recently is
chlorpyrifos, from the organophosphate chemical family, a relatively
inexpensive and widely used pesticide. A large body of research from the
EPA and the National Institutes of Health has shown that when pregnant women are exposed to chlorpyrifos, their children exhibit lower
IQ scores, weaker mental development, and increased rates of ADHD.[27]
You might also find it frightening to learn that in World War II, the
German military developed organophosphates as neurotoxins, meaning they were used in chemical warfare! Granted, higher doses were used
compared to what's commonly used to kill pests on crops today, but I
don't want even a trace of neurotoxins on my kids' food. Chlorpyrifos is
heavily used on foods that we eat frequently, like corn, nuts, soybeans,
wheat, fruits, and vegetables. In the United States, millions of pounds of
it are sprayed onto our food supply each year. But if you live in California
or Hawaii, there's good news—chlorpyrifos is banned there, following
studies in 2017 and 2018 showing exposure caused anxiety, hyperactivity,
and learning problems in rats at lower doses than previously tested in
humans. New York plans to phase them out too.[28]

Because there are quite a few dangers lurking in conventionally grown produce, it's crucial to try to eat organic produce as much as possible, and for children, it's even more important. The most prevalent way we are exposed to pesticides is through food we consume. Children are even more susceptible to the health effects because they eat more pound for pound in relation to what adults eat.[29] Exposure during infancy and childhood can be especially harmful because the health effects can interfere with important body systems as they're developing. Insecticides are a particular kind of pesticide that is used specifically to kill insects. Though these chemicals rarely cause illness, these insecticides "have the potential to cause long-term damage to the brain and nervous system, which are rapidly growing...during early childhood."[30] And guess where a lot of that insecticide exposure is found? In the foods these children eat frequently, like apples (whole apples, but also applesauce and apple juice), popcorn, grapes, and peaches. Thousands of children that the EWG studied consumed more insecticides than what's considered safe by federal standards, and more than half received that unsafe dose *just* from apple products. So for a lot of kids, a *conventional* apple a day might *not* keep the doctor away.

Conventional farmers can also spray crops with strong chemical-laden weed and insect killers and use hormones in livestock, which gets into our meat and dairy. Luckily, studies also show that eating organic just for several days can greatly reduce levels of pesticides in our bodies.[31] Not all fruits and vegetables have the same level of exposure to pesticides, so depending on which type of produce you're shopping for, in some cases—like the Dirty Dozen, which I'll explain below—you should always buy organic.

Are organic foods more nutritious?

There has been some debate about whether organic food really is more nutritious, and both health experts and consumers have been arguing about it for some time. A 2012 study in the *Annals of Internal Medicine* detailed the work of researchers at Stanford University who evaluated nearly 250 studies comparing the nutrients of organic versus nonorganic foods.[32] The researchers found very little discernible difference in nutritional value, though they did find a 30 percent lower pesticide residue in organic produce. The researchers claimed that since the pesticide levels were within allowable safety limits, it wasn't yet clear what the implications were for health. But some research has shown that in addition to being contaminated with fewer pesticides, nitrates, and heavy metals, organic produce also contains significantly more vitamin C, iron, and magnesium than nonorganic.[33] In 2014, in response to the Stanford study that sparked much controversy, a group of scientists based in Europe analyzed data from over 340 studies and published their findings in the *British Journal of Nutrition.* They concluded that organic fruits and vegetables deliver between 20 and 40 percent more antioxidant compounds, like flavonoids or carotenoids, and are believed to protect cells from the damage that can lead to aging or even cancer.[34] They also determined that organic crops had about 50 percent more anthocyanins and flavonols as compared to conventional crops. Anthocyanins are compounds that give fruits and vegetables, such as blueberries, their blue, purple, and red hues, and consuming them is linked to a host of health benefits, such as reducing inflammation. Flavonols are a group of compounds found in foods and beverages like tea, cocoa, apples, and grapes; they are known to contribute to healthy circulation and overall health.[35]

In 2016, another large study that combined data from over two hundred studies was published in the *British Journal of Nutrition*, further contributing to the growing evidence that organic food packs a more significant nutritional punch. That study found that organic meat and dairy contained about 50 percent more omega-3 fatty acids.[36]

Though some health experts and consumers will continue to argue about whether the health benefits of organic food are significant enough to justify the added cost, for me, the benefits are clear, especially when it comes to buying organic produce.

Slightly greener organic produce shopping

Personally, I like to buy organic whenever I can. As I've explained in this chapter, the benefits from organics are twofold: fewer chemicals *and* potentially more nutrients. However, I also understand that organic products are not always available or affordable. That's no problem—it's possible to shop organic on a budget. One way to do that is to use the EWG's Clean 15 and Dirty Dozen lists as a reference. The Dirty Dozen is the EWG's trademarked term for the twelve crops that farmers usually use the most pesticides on. The Clean 15 is another trademarked term to describe the fifteen crops with the lowest amount of pesticide residue. (The list is updated every year, so check the EWG's website periodically to look for changes.)

The Clean 15[37]

Avocados	Onions	Eggplant	Cantaloupe	Cabbage
Sweet corn	Papaya	Asparagus	Broccoli	Honeydew Melon
Pineapple	Frozen Sweet Peas	Cauliflower	Mushrooms	Kiwi

The Dirty Dozen[38]

Strawberries	Nectarines	Peaches	Tomatoes
Spinach	Apples	Cherries	Celery
Kale	Grapes	Pears	Potatoes

The truth about farmers markets and health food stores

I often find that clients assume foods found in certain stores are organic without verifying individual products. They shop at Whole Foods or their local farmers market and say, "All their food is organic, right?" Nope. Not necessarily. Some consumers give those natural food stores way more credit than they deserve, assuming that every product on their shelves has been carefully checked for health and safety. In most cases, they haven't. For example, one of my friends found an electrolyte powder at her local health store in the Bay Area that she loved. "It tastes like grape-flavored Kool-Aid!" she told me. She assumed that since she bought it at her local health food store, it was safe—even organic. Plus there were other labels on the plastic bottle that made her trust the electrolyte product, terms like *natural*, *vegan*, and *gluten-free*. She read those words and thought it meant "safe."

This is a perfect example of *greenwashing*. Greenwashing is when companies design their packaging so a product *looks* like it's good for you (or for the environment). However, this client did admit shock at how delicious the flavor was. (If it feels too good to be true, it probably is!) I asked her to share the label with me and saw the words *natural flavors* listed in the ingredients. I explained that the term *natural flavors* means that the flavor originated from a natural source but that it can have many chemicals added to it after the fact. We'll dig deeper into how the natural and artificial flavors industry works later in the chapter. My client tossed out the electrolyte product and realized that you can't assume a product is safe just because you bought it in a certain store.

What about local farmers markets? Those sell organic foods, right? Once again, you need to do your research. In 2017, CBC News in Ontario, Canada, sent an undercover team to investigate farmers markets to see where their produce came from. They found five different vendors who *claimed* to be selling organic produce they'd grown themselves, when in fact, they hadn't grown the foods at all. In a few cases, the sellers had purchased the produce from a wholesale market.[39] The *New York Times* reported a similar story in 2010, where an investigation by a Los Angeles NBC affiliate found that some local farmers market produce actually came from warehouses and commercial (not organic) farms.[40] The lesson here? Always ask questions about the food you buy. Where was it grown? How was it cared for?

FARMERS MARKET TIPS

Before you buy produce at a farmers market, ask these questions:

→ Where was the food grown?

→ When was it picked?

→ What was used on the crops to control pests?

If the sellers are at all wary of answering any of the above questions, reconsider buying from that vendor.

What's behind the "natural" label

Now let's consider what happens when you see the term *natural* on a food product. What does that term tell you? Here's the hard truth. The word *natural* is utterly meaningless on food labels, because the FDA doesn't regulate it and it has no official definition, leaving companies with the power to define it however they please. When a food is labeled "natural," it simply means that product is natural according to the company's definition. That's right: the people who manufacture and profit from that product get to decide what "natural" means to them. Are they being transparent and truthful? It's hard to tell. Another issue: research has found that when consumers see the term *natural* on a product label, they believe it holds significance. In fact, a 2015 survey found that 60 percent of consumers thought that the term *natural* on packaged foods meant that those items were made with no toxic pesticides, no artificial colors or ingredients, and no GMOs.[41] But it's quite possible that those foods *do* have GMOs, chemicals, additives, and other dangerous ingredients. According to a survey from Consumer Reports, consumers are more likely to buy foods that are labeled "natural" (this term isn't regulated) over ones that are labeled "organic" (this term *is* highly regulated by the FDA).[42]

My trick for remembering this information is to say, "Natural is not regulated and not necessarily healthy." From now on, just look at labels that say "natural" the same way that you would the word *delicious*. It's subjective.

Of course, some companies aren't abusing trust with this label, but others add the term *natural* to their packaging because they think it might convince you to buy their product. One of the first things my clients say to me is, "What? How can companies put 'natural' on a label if it's meaningless? And why doesn't the FDA regulate it?" If you feel frustrated that you've been loading your grocery cart with "all natural" products, know that you're not alone. According to a report by the *Washington Post* citing data from the market research firm Nielsen, foods labeled "natural" made up $40.7 billion in sales in 2013.[43] Many consumers have a sense of false trust in that label.

> "Natural" = not regulated, not necessarily healthy.

Other label reading tips

Another tricky term, *pesticide-free*, is not regulated either. This is a problem, considering that a 2018 Consumer Reports survey found that 48 percent of respondents prioritize looking for a "pesticide-free" label.[44] Ingredient lists are not required from smaller companies, and those with lower annual sales are exempt from listing their ingredients. If possible, look for items that have ingredient labels, and be sure to ask how the product was made if you are at a farmers market.

Another trick I like to share with clients when label sleuthing: ingredients are listed in order from the largest percentage to the smallest. For example, if you look at a box of cereal and the ingredients read sugar, wheat, and dried strawberries, you might think, *Breakfast of champions!* You might call me up and say, "This cereal has ingredients I can spell and pronounce. High-five me, Tonya!" But I will tell you to toss that box of cereal in the trash can. (Or just eat it by the handful like a dessert for special occasions.) Because the majority of that cereal is made up of good, old-fashioned sugar. The wheat and the strawberries are just a vehicle for funneling sugar into your mouth! Another challenge? There are over sixty different names for sugar, and cereals—as well as other foods—often contain several different types of sugar. While some of these aliases for sugar are fairly obvious (like cane sugar, for example), others are downright tricky to spot (like maltodextrin). This is when it's helpful to remember the 80/20 rule. I'm not saying don't ever eat cereal. I'm also not saying you need to eliminate sugar or banish iced cinnamon rolls from your diet for the rest of your life. Just try to make safe and healthy choices 80 percent of the time. You don't need to memorize all sixty different names for sugar. But if you want to learn the most common ones you'll see on the label, here is your chance!

OTHER NAMES FOR SUGAR

Ingredients (some not listed below) that end in the word *sugar*

Ingredients that have an *-ose* at the end of the name, like dextrose, maltose, or fructose

Agave	Glucose
Agave nectar	Glucose solids
Barley malt	Glucose syrup
Blackstrap molasses	Golden syrup
Cane juice	High fructose corn syrup
Cane juice solids	Honey
Cane juice crystals	Lactose
Cane syrup	Maltose
Carob syrup	Malt sugar
Corn syrup	Malt syrup
Corn syrup solids	Maple syrup
Crystalline fructose	Molasses
Dextrose	Muscovado
Dehydrated cane juice	Nectar
Evaporated cane juice	Panocha
Evaporated cane syrup	Refiners' syrup
Evaporated sugar cane	Sorghum
Fructose	Sorghum syrup
Fruit juice concentrate	Sucanat
Galactose	Sucrose
Glazing sugar	

The problem with hidden sugars

This isn't a diet book, so we won't go into nutrition too in-depth, but it's worth briefly talking about sugar. Consuming natural sugar that occurs in whole foods, like strawberries, is fine, but when you start to consume too many added sugars—that is, additional sugars that food manufacturers add to the product to make it taste better or to length the shelf life—that is when the health problems start to occur. Yet sugar is found in the majority of our foods and drinks and in the large majority of our processed foods. The typical American consumes about twenty-two teaspoons of added sugar per day. A man's recommended daily intake is around nine teaspoons per day, and a woman's is about six.[45] Sugar often hides behind other names and is found in some surprising foods you might even think of as healthy, like yogurt and salad dressings.

With unwanted health effects such as metabolic syndrome, insulin resistance, diabetes, weight gain, and even links to cancer, added sugar is something we should avoid as much as possible.[46] A study published in 2014 in *JAMA Internal Medicine* found an association between a diet high in added sugar and a greater risk of dying from heart disease.[47] In that study, people who consumed 17 to 21 percent of their calories from added sugar had a 38 percent higher risk of dying from cardiovascular disease compared to those who consumed 8 percent of their diet as added sugar. Consuming too much added sugar can also increase blood pressure, raise chronic inflammation, and cause weight gain, diabetes, and fatty liver disease, which are all linked to an increase in heart attack and stroke risk.[48]

When you're reading the ingredients in your food, look out for ones that end in *-ose*, such as dextrose, maltose, or sucrose, and anything that ends in the words *sugar* or *syrup*. Even an organic sugary treat can be important to avoid. While there are benefits to eating an organic versus a nonorganic treat, you still need to read your labels carefully. A cookie is still a cookie.

REDUCE SUGAR INTAKE

→ Avoid ingredients that end in the word *sugar*.

→ Avoid ingredients that end in -ose, like dextrose, maltose, and sucrose.

→ See the Resources section for a full list of other names for sugar.

The bottom line

While it's tempting to fall for alluring packages that promise to deliver healthy food that tastes great, many of the food products that *look* healthy and safe simply aren't. Add to this the fact that we are faced with an overwhelming number of food product options when we arrive at the grocery store, and it's a serious challenge to know how to buy safe and healthy products. Now you know a bit more about how to read labels more carefully and what the different terms and designations mean. In the next chapter, we'll cover *specific* ingredients to avoid in food, and in no time, you'll breeze through the grocery aisles and know exactly what to look for. Together we will review ten different ingredients in food that I suggest you avoid. We've already covered one—hidden sugars. But I promise, it won't all be kale and brussels sprouts on this journey. There will be sweets in your future.

5

"Safe" Ingredients to Avoid

Today, about 60 percent of the foods Americans eat are processed, and diet-related illnesses have become the leading cause of mortality in this country.[1] And as the number of chemicals we're exposed to grows daily, it's more important than ever before to pay attention to what's in our food. There are over ten thousand different substances like emulsifiers, preservatives, color, and flavoring added to processed food to keep it fresh or to improve its texture, taste, or appearance.[2] In his popular book *Food Rules*, Michael Pollan said, "Don't eat anything your great-grandmother wouldn't recognize as food."[3] This is excellent advice. One of the best ways we can avoid harmful ingredients in our diets is by not eating processed foods in the first place! Cooking at home and consuming fresh, whole foods should always be the goal. But of course we want to eat occasional snacks, treats, and desserts; it is the *Slightly*

Greener Method after all. In this chapter, I will highlight ten ingredients to avoid in food. As always, I will remind you to *remember your why* as you read, as you don't have to eliminate every single ingredient right away. It's better to start with one or two and build from there.

What *are* processed foods, really?

I doubt I'm the first to tell you to avoid processed foods. But what *are* they exactly, and what health problems do they cause? You might think of processed food as anything that comes in a can, a bag, or a box, which is true. But more broadly, processing means taking any fresh food (like corn) and turning it into a food product (like corn chips). Different food processing methods include freezing, canning, heating, fermenting, cooking, packaging, pasteurizing—anything that transforms a whole food into a food "product," which could just mean putting it into a package. When food is processed, it's often combined with additives that boost taste, like sugar, salt, and oil, or preservatives to help keep it fresh. This is why processed foods taste so good!

But processing food isn't new. Human beings have been adding things to food to extend shelf life, boost flavor, and increase convenience for centuries, like salting bacon or pickling food with vinegar. It makes food options cheaper, more convenient, longer lasting, better tasting, but not always healthier.

Processed food is also exposed to what are called *indirect additives*—substances like plastics and oils in packaging or containers that can leach into the food itself. Food can also come into contact with chemicals or contaminants during processing, storage, and transportation.

An example of an indirect additive is the phthalates that have been found in the powdered cheese mixes of macaroni and cheese products. Phthalates are endocrine disrupting chemicals that have been banned in products like plastic teething rings for babies. A study published by the Coalition for Safer Food Processing and Packaging found that of thirty different samples of cheese products tested, including sliced as well as packaged cheese—such as cottage cheese—in addition to the powdered cheese mixes, twenty-nine of them contained phthalates.[4] In this case, the phthalates aren't a direct ingredient or additive in the food product. Instead, they are likely an indirect result of the packaging, storage, or shipping process. In this particular study, there were ten different phthalates found, with the highest concentrations in the powdered cheese. The phthalates that were found can cause health issues like reproductive, respiratory, and neurobehavioral issues, which means cognitive, behavioral, or emotional challenges. And according to the Environmental Defense Fund (EDF), every chemical in the phthalate class that has been tested for health effects has been found to have an associated health risk. The EDF has noted that despite that, nearly half of the FDA-approved chemicals in the phthalate category don't have any safety data published on them at all.

Fast food consumption is another method for phthalate exposure through food. A 2016 study found that people who frequently eat fast food had as much as 40 percent more phthalates in their urine. The author of that particular study cited PVC tubing, food packaging, and vinyl gloves as the possible sources.[5] The takeaway here? Phthalates are in packaged foods, and we *know* they're bad. To what extent remains a bit unclear, but we do know that minimizing our exposure to takeout and packaged foods is the best idea.

But don't worry. You don't have to live without the occasional chips, cookie, or frozen pizza. We're only human after all. In many cases, it's easy to make a homemade version yourself, and there are certainly some processed foods that are better than others.

A little history on food preservation

In addition to understanding what the heck processed foods really are, I think it's also interesting to note *how* and *why* our food industry creates so much processed food in the first place. Like many innovations, food processing and packaging started with good intentions. Fun fact: in 1809, a French chef named Nicolas Appert invented the method of preserving food by putting it in completely airtight containers. At the time, France's army was spread out all over Europe, and as soldiers traveled, their food spoiled. Appert's invention came to the rescue. Thus began food processing as we know it.

Over the coming years, food processing became more popular as new methods were developed and processed foods became cheaper to make. World War I brought on new methods of processing, like commercially sold canned and frozen foods in the 1920s. In the 1950s, processed foods became mass distributed, and ready-to-eat meals were marketed as a way to liberate women from cooking at home. At that time, the food industry launched a campaign telling women they could save time by buying packaged foods. This began a sweeping movement with the message "Liberate yourself from the stove!" And as women in particular were increasingly marketed packaged foods as a way to simplify their lives, they were given ever more options from which to choose. The 1950s saw the birth of the chicken nugget (1963),[6] high fructose corn syrup (1967),[7] and Tang (1959).[8] In the 1960s, we saw the introduction of Tab[9] and Diet Pepsi, as well as Pringles[10] and Gatorade.[11] And in the 1970s, the FDA banned food coloring FD&C Red No. 2 because studies showed that it might cause cancer, and the red M&Ms disappeared for eleven years.[12]

In the 1980s, the food industry continued to further develop its range of packaged food offerings and ingredients: the artificial sweetener aspartame was approved by the FDA, the USDA announced that ketchup counted as a vegetable in a school lunch[13]. In the 1990s, Americans started consuming huge amounts of caloric sweeteners.[14] But there was one piece of good news: the 1990 Nutrition Labeling and Education Act stated that all packaged foods must have standard nutrition labeling.[15] Today, there are over ten thousand chemicals and additives allowed to be added to foods,[16] many of which are linked to hormone disruption and other health effects, of which the cumulative and synergistic effects are unknown.[17]

With each passing year since Appert first figured out how to make food last longer by placing it in a sealed container, the idea that making food last longer and taste better—even at the cost of using chemicals and preservatives to do so—drove much of food and packaging development. But as we now well know, just because a Twinkie is cheap to make, tastes delicious, and seemingly lasts forever doesn't make it a good food choice.

How additives get into our food

OK, so our food is filled with things that make it cheaper, better tasting, and longer lasting. But how do additives in food get from the chemistry lab to our plates? When a company wants to include food additives in its product, it has two choices. Option one is formal FDA approval—a process that can take years, even decades. So it's not surprising that most companies choose a much faster alternative route. If the company would like, it can choose to have its food additive declared "generally recognized as safe," or GRAS. To be deemed GRAS, the company *itself* decides that what it's adding to the food is safe. Notifying the FDA is completely voluntary. Yes, you read that right: companies do not have to inform the FDA about additives used.[18]

According to a 2016 survey by the Consumer Reports National Research Center, the term GRAS can be misleading for consumers: 77 percent of people surveyed believed that GRAS meant the FDA had evaluated the ingredient and found it to be safe.[19] The survey also found that 66 percent of respondents believed the FDA regularly monitors the safety and use of GRAS ingredients But both of these statements are false. Originally, in 1958, the GRAS designation was established by a law that required companies to prove that their prospective ingredients were safe. The GRAS exception was meant to be just that—an exception for common household ingredients like baking soda or vinegar that were in wide use and known to be safe. But in 1997, the FDA introduced a new rule that allowed companies to decide for themselves whether or not their ingredients were GRAS, and now we have what is essentially a loophole for companies, without action taken by the FDA. Watchdog groups like the Government Accountability Office and the Center for Food Safety have proposed several recommendations to the FDA to improve the safety oversight of chemicals in our food, like excluding novel chemicals or risky substances from being declared GRAS, making GRAS designations mandatory and public, and ensuring the reviews are only executed by independent, unbiased experts, but none of these suggestions have been adopted by the FDA.

There are estimated to be over one thousand GRAS substances in which the designations were made without any heads-up to the FDA. And there are thought to be thousands of chemicals for which the oversight and safety review process was minimal.[20]

When it comes to additives, the term *natural* doesn't necessarily mean safe, just as we have seen with other uses of the term *natural* on food labels. For example, safrole, which occurs naturally in sassafras and sweet basil, is a natural additive that used to be added to flavor root beer, until it was found to be carcinogenic.[21] It's important to point out that you don't want to necessarily replace one artificial additive with a natural one and assume it's better.

The bottom line: there are a significant number of chemicals in processed foods that simply haven't been adequately tested for the safety of human consumption.

As we dig into each of the ingredients to avoid in this chapter, you will notice that they have been called "safe" by the FDA or deemed GRAS, but there has been controversy swirling around them, in some cases for a very long time. So I like to err on the side of caution, because in some cases, additives are often widely used before they are discovered to be harmful. The *good news* is that consumers are beginning to demand more transparency, and as a result, companies are responding. I've researched the most commonly used ingredients that I recommend you avoid. Together we will go through each one, and I will explain why you should avoid them and where you will find them.

1. Natural flavors

A food's particular taste is largely the result of the volatile chemicals in the food. The chemicals that give a food its smell are very important, as to our brains, the way a food tastes is a blend of the food's taste, smell, and touch combined into one sensation.[22] The particular mixture of chemicals that makes up the smell in foods is called flavor.

Many clients I work with adore canned sparkling water. Who doesn't? The tingling bubbles, the tasty natural flavors—what's not to love? But I'm sad to report that these zero-calorie drinks aren't as innocent as advertised. The "natural" flavors responsible for that orange or black cherry taste can be made up of dozens of different chemicals. The FDA states that a natural flavor is "a substance extracted, distilled, or similarly derived from plant or animal matter, either as is or after it has been roasted, heated, or fermented, and whose function is for flavor, not nutrition."[23] According to the EWG, "natural flavor" is the fourth most common ingredient in their list of over eighty thousand foods, behind salt, sugar, and water.[24]

So should you avoid natural flavors? For me, the short answer is yes. The ingredients in natural flavors aren't required to be disclosed, as they are considered trade secrets. For that reason alone, I would definitely recommend avoiding natural flavors as much as possible. Legally, natural flavors can include over one hundred different chemicals in addition to their original flavor source. Those chemicals can include preservatives, solvents, and other additives. Because these formulas are considered to be proprietary, food and beverage manufacturers aren't required to disclose where these additives come from, including whether they're derived from natural or synthetic sources. As long as the original flavoring source comes from a plant or animal, it is classified as a natural flavor. If you are following a special diet or have food allergies or sensitivities, you may want to contact the company to see if they'll disclose the ingredients. You may also want to do this if you're a vegetarian or a vegan, because some of the ingredients that make up natural flavors may be animal derived, but you wouldn't know it from what's on the label.

2. Artificial flavors

Artificial flavors are created in a laboratory by trained professionals known as flavorists or flavor chemists, and they spend significant scientific engineering and design effort to create widely appealing flavors. An artificial flavor can be made up of any combination of the nearly seven hundred FDA-allowed flavoring chemicals or food additives that have been deemed GRAS.[25] It can also be comprised of one of the two thousand other chemicals sanctioned not by the FDA but by the Flavor and Extract Manufacturers Association of the United States.

In some cases, the chemical mixtures of artificial flavors are simpler as they tend to be composed of fewer chemicals than those of natural flavors, which can contain hundreds of chemicals.[26] The flavor industry says that artificial flavors adhere to a more rigorous set of safety measures. But the reality is that neither are entirely thorough or safe. For those reasons, I steer clear of both as often as possible! Artificial flavors are any flavors that are not defined as natural, even if they have the exact same chemical composition as flavors isolated directly from nature.[27] The distinction between artificial and natural is pegged to the original source of the flavor, not its safety.

3. High fructose corn syrup

High fructose corn syrup (HFCS) is an ingredient found in many processed foods, such as cookies, crackers, chips, cereals, salad dressings, condiments, fruit juices, and sodas and even in medication and some children's vitamins. It is linked to health effects such as diabetes, wrinkling of the skin, obesity, collagen damage, metabolic syndrome, increased cellulite, hypertension, accelerated aging, and an increased cancer risk. It was originally developed in 1957, when it was created to replace expensive cane sugar with a cheaper sweetener made from corn.[28] In the 1970s, HFCS started to gain traction in the market, but at that time, it only represented less than 1 percent of all caloric sweeteners. Caloric sweeteners (also known as nutritive sweeteners) provide energy in the form of carbohydrates.[29] These also include other added sugars such as honey, molasses, cane sugar, or maple syrup. But by 2004, the use of HFCS had ballooned to 42 percent of all caloric sweeteners.

There is some debate on whether or not HFCS is linked to weight gain, but a study published in the *American Journal of Clinical Nutrition* found that the body rapidly converts fructose into fat.[30] When you eat a starchy food like rice, your body breaks it down into glucose, which is easily transported throughout the body and used for energy. However, table sugar and HFCS contain 50 percent glucose and 50 percent fructose, which is metabolized differently.[31] This is different from the natural fructose you consume from fresh fruit, which is good for you and nearly impossible to consume in excess.[32] But when your body consumes excess processed fructose, it then has to convert it into glucose, glycogen (which is stored as carbohydrates), or fat before your body can use it as energy.[33] Add to that the fact that HFCS doesn't have any nutritional value at all, and you have plenty of reasons to avoid it.

HFCS can also be contaminated with other substances. In fact, one particular study published in the journal *Environmental Health* found that half of all the commercial HFCS samples tested were found to be contaminated with mercury.[34] Mercury is a known neurotoxin. In another study, the Institute for Agriculture and Trade Policy tested popular foods that contain HFCS for the presence of mercury. Of fifty-five samples tested, they found detectable levels of mercury in 31 percent of them.[35] This contamination is a result of the production process, where the HFCS has been made using mercury-grade caustic soda. Mercury exposure can cause issues such as loss of IQ points as well as decreased performance in tests involving memory, attention, language, and even spatial cognition. Kidney damage and heart function alteration have also been reported.[36]

We can't completely eliminate our exposure to mercury—we breathe it in from industrial pollution in the air, for example—but we can likely reduce our overall exposure just by avoiding HFCS in processed foods.

For me, there are plenty of reasons not to consume HFCS. I'm clear on my decision: I'm avoiding it for my family and recommend that you do too.

HOW TO AVOID HFCS

→ Do not purchase foods with HFCS on the label.

→ Eat fast food and restaurant food less often.

→ Eat organic foods as much as possible.

→ Avoid drinking soda and commercially made fruit juice.

→ Cook at home with whole foods as much as possible.

---

4. Monosodium glutamate

Monosodium glutamate (MSG) is the most widely used food additive in the world. It's found in many different processed foods, including chips, salad dressings, sauces, commercial soups, and even spices. When I bring it up, people usually say, "Oh my gosh, MSG, right— Chinese food." Which is true—MSG is found in a lot of takeout and restaurant foods. But clients are shocked to learn that MSG is also in so many of the packaged foods we eat every day. Based on what I've seen in the research as well as the results I've seen in my family—and in my clients—I don't think MSG gets the attention it deserves. Some people are quite sensitive to it, exhibiting headaches, heart palpitations, tingling feelings, or face tightening after consuming it. Though MSG has been declared GRAS, it has been linked to health problems like obesity and attention issues.

Dr. Russell Blaylock, author of *Excitotoxins: The Taste That Kills*, believes MSG can damage children's brain health by affecting the development of the nervous system to the point that they may have learning and emotional difficulties years later.[37] According to Dr. Blaylock, when neurons—nerve cells in the brain that are the building blocks of the nervous system—are exposed to MSG, they become overexcited and quickly fire off impulses until they reach a state of extreme exhaustion. Their job is to transmit information to the other nerve cells, but instead, several hours after the MSG exposure, these neurons die off, as if they were excited to death. This is why MSG is known as an *excitotoxin*, a term coined by Dr. Blaylock.

Numerous studies have also revealed that feeding MSG to pregnant animals produced a type of learning difficulty similar to ADHD. Their offspring didn't have noticeable differences in simple learning but showed profound differences when it came to learning more complex things, along with a decrease in important neurotransmitters in the forebrain.[38] If you're familiar with ADHD, you may be familiar with the prefrontal cortex, which is located in the frontal lobe. This part of the brain plays a role in self-regulation (behavior and making good choices), memory, language and speech, mood, and social behavior. It's also responsible for executive function skills, which include time management, multitasking, and the ability to start tasks.

MSG has also been linked to obesity. Researchers have found that an injury to the part of the brain called the hypothalamus can cause animals to become obese, and MSG has been discovered to cause lesions there.[39] The hypothalamus regulates hormones as well as critical body functions like heart rate, sleep cycles, weight, and appetite. MSG also shuts off leptin, the hormone that tells us we're full.[40] Leptin enters the brain and acts on neurons in the hypothalamus to let the brain know that the body has had enough food, suppressing appetite. But animal studies have shown that MSG suppresses leptin, causing them to overeat because they don't get that "stop, you're full!" signal.

It can be tough to find processed foods that are truly MSG-free. It's heavily used in restaurant food, and there are over forty common food ingredients that *contain* MSG. You can also find MSG in medications and even in vitamins (in the ingredients that bind and fill them). If you do choose MSG as an ingredient to avoid, beware of the fine print. For example, a soup may be labeled as containing "no MSG," but then you may see a little symbol like this (†) following it, which indicates that there *is* MSG in that food, even though it's not listed on the label. But when you look at the back of the label you might see "except for that which occurs naturally in hydrolyzed wheat protein." Sneaky, right? What that label is saying is that while MSG itself was not technically added to the product, other ingredients that naturally contain MSG have been added, so MSG exposure is possible. The synthetic version of MSG may be more potent, but people who are sensitive to MSG tend to react to both, as the body doesn't distinguish between the source of the MSG but rather the potency.[41] Be sure to carefully check your labels for all the ingredients. It's common to find foods that have several sources of MSG listed.

There is a lot of debate surrounding MSG, but for all the reasons stated above, I recommend that you avoid it. There is also evidence of children's behavior improving and ADHD symptoms lessening when MSG is removed from the diet, and I've seen it in my own family. MSG is found in a lot of processed foods and things that really aren't good for us anyway, so it can't hurt to avoid it!

How to avoid MSG

Common MSG ingredients you'll see listed on the label:
Hydrolyzed vegetable protein

Textured vegetable protein

Yeast extract or autolyzed yeast

*MSG may also be hiding under the term *natural flavors*

These ingredients *always* contain MSG:
Glutamic acid

Glutamate

Monosodium glutamate

Calcium caseinate

Sodium caseinate

Yeast extract

Yeast food

Yeast nutrient

Autolyzed yeast

Gelatin

Textured protein

Soy protein isolate

Whey protein/whey protein isolate

Anything with the words "protein," "hydrolyzed," "hydrolyzed
      protein," or "protein fortified"

Anything with the words "enzyme," "enzyme modified," or
      "fermented"

These ingredients *often* contain MSG:

Carrageenan

Bouillon and broth

Stock

Natural flavors (natural beef, pork, or chicken flavoring)

Maltodextrin

Barley malt/malted barley

Malt extract

Citric acid, citrate

Pectin

Protease

Soy sauce

Soy sauce extract

Seasonings (including Lawry's and Accent)

These ingredients may cause reactions in those who are sensitive to MSG due to naturally occurring MSG within them:[42]

Cornstarch

Corn syrup/HFCS

Corn syrup solids

Rice syrup

Brown rice syrup

Dextrose

Fructose

Spices

Caramel coloring or flavoring

Soy lecithin

Gums (guar, vegetable, xanthan)

Modified food starch

Lipolyzed butter fat

Annatto

Vinegar

Balsamic vinegar

Milk powder

Reduced fat milk (skim, 1%, 2%)

Most things "low fat" or "no fat"

Anything "vitamin enriched"

Anything "pasteurized"

Certain amino acid chelates (Citrate, aspartate, and glutamate are
    used as chelating agents with mineral supplements.)

Also look for MSG in these items:

Gel caps for vitamins or supplements, if made from animal gelatin
or hydrolyzed vegetable protein

Vitamins and medications that contain binders and fillers (be on the
lookout for cornstarch, yeast, dextrose, and amino acids created
from soy, yeast, and dairy)

Toothpastes (those that contain carrageenan)

Stevia packets (stevia is a great sweeter on its own, but when it's
packaged into packets, it's mixed with maltodextrin, which may
contain MSG)

Shampoos, cosmetics (hydrolyzed proteins are common)

5. Carrageenan

Carrageenan is an extract from red seaweed, otherwise known as Irish
moss, and it has been used in foods for centuries.[43] It's used in food as
an emulsifier, a substance that combines ingredients and helps a mixture retain its texture. Carrageenan is commonly used to improve the
texture of ice cream, yogurt, and cottage cheese as well as dairy-free
products (like coconut milk), coffee creamers, and infant formulas.
Because it is derived from seaweed, it has long been considered safe
and is frequently found in organic or "healthy" brands. What doesn't
sound healthy about *seaweed?*

Unfortunately, carrageenan has been linked to health problems like
chronic colitis, belly bloat, inflammation, spastic colon, weight gain,
diabetes, glucose intolerance, and inflammatory bowel disease.[44] Other

studies have found a connection that suggest carrageenan in the human diet may contribute to the development of diabetes, but the results aren't conclusive.[45] Studies have revealed that carrageenan is inflammatory to the digestive tract.[46] In fact, researchers have used injectable carrageenan to cause inflammation in tissues in animal testing just so that they can test the anti-inflammatory properties of new drugs.[47]

6. Artificial sweeteners

AVOID THESE ARTIFICIAL SWEETENERS

→ Aspartame (NutraSweet, Equal)

→ Acesulfame potassium (acesulfame K, Ace K)

→ Neotame

→ Saccharin (Sweet 'N Low, Sweet Twin)

→ Sucralose (Splenda, NatraTaste Gold)

SAFER SWEETENERS

→ Raw honey

→ Dates, date puree

→ Coconut sugar

→ Grade B maple syrup

→ Brown rice syrup

→ Yacon syrup

Six artificial sweeteners approved for use in the United States include:

aspartame, sucralose, acesulfame potassium (or acesulfame K), advantame, neotame, and saccharin. There is still some debate about the dangers of artificial sweeteners, but just like HFCS, they are often found in foods that aren't good for you anyway.

These sweeteners are often touted as tools for weight loss and are found in "diet" and "sugar-free" foods such as Jell-O, flavored water, and even chewing gum. One of the ironic health effects of artificial sweeteners is that they can cause weight gain! The 2008 San Antonio Heart Study found that those who drank more than twenty-one diet drinks per week were twice as likely to become overweight or obese as people who didn't drink diet soda.[48] Drinking regular soda also increased the risk for obesity, but what was most surprising was the fact that the study participants who drank *diet* soda had an even *higher* increase in obesity risk. For those who drank regular soft drinks, the risk of becoming overweight or obese was 32.8 percent for those who consumed one to two cans each day. For those who drank diet soft drinks, the risk of becoming overweight or obese was 54.5 percent for one to two cans each day.

The lead researcher from that study also found a 41 percent increase in risk of becoming overweight for every can or bottle of diet soft drink a person consumes each day. The reason? Artificial sweeteners turn on what's called the *cephalic response*, because our modern brains have never tasted something so sweet; artificial sweeteners are four hundred to six hundred times sweeter than regular table sugar. Even something as seemingly natural as stevia has proven to cause the cephalic response! The cephalic response is the result of our body's programming to execute a "biological cascade" of reactions when we taste something that sweet. The body releases insulin (which stores sugar in the bloodstream) and gets ready for the carbohydrates it thinks it is about to receive, but if it doesn't get the carbohydrates, blood sugar drops and creates an urge for those expected calories. This typically causes us to overeat because the stomach didn't get what it was expecting. Your stomach says: *feed me!* Insulin is released whether or not carbohydrates are received by the body, and this release of insulin tells the body to store fat.

Researchers have found that even just swishing diet soda around in the mouth and then spitting out causes the cephalic response.[49] Fat cells have "key codes" that open them: the glycemic index of a food and insulin. When a fat cell is triggered, it opens up and lets fat in, then the fat cells get bigger and start dividing. When you drink diet soda, the cephalic response is activated, releasing insulin. Fat cells have now been allowed to open up because the insulin unlocked them. The same is true for all artificial sweeteners and foods that are labeled "sugar-free" or "zero calorie." Consuming foods and drinks that do not contain calories or sugar may actually make it almost impossible to lose weight!

Research has also found a newly discovered way in which artificial sweeteners can cause weight gain: they disrupt the gut flora.[50] Gut microbes play an important role in overall health as well as in obesity. Scientists used to believe that our billions of microscopic gut bacteria were primarily significant for digestion, but new evidence reveals that our gut bacteria can also influence the way we store fat, how glucose levels are stabilized in the blood, and how we react to the hormones that signal hunger and fullness.[51] Rodent studies and recent studies on twins have revealed a less diverse microflora in those who are obese, and those studies showed that lean people tended to have a wider variety of microbes that specialized in breaking down plant starches and fibers into molecules that the body could more easily use as an energy source. An alteration of gut flora can also disrupt pathways in the body that are responsible for sugar transport throughout the body, which could lead to glucose intolerance, a precursor to type 2 diabetes, even in healthy individuals. Glucose intolerance can also cause weight gain, as the excess sugars circulating through the blood typically end up being stored in fat cells.

So if you find yourself just having to have a soda, I recommend regular soda instead of the diet version. There are also some other great options—healthy carbonated drinks that give you the satisfaction of a refreshing bubbly drink without the harmful chemicals or added sugar. For example, I love the brand Spindrift, which makes healthy carbonated water mixed with real fruit juice. Olipop is another great beverage brand that makes delicious versions of root beer and cola with safe, clinically backed ingredients. I also like to make my own carbonated beverages using a SodaStream. If you're not familiar, a SodaStream is an at-home sparkling water maker. You simply use your own filter to create carbonated water, add a fresh slice of lemon, and—I swear—it tastes almost exactly like Sprite! If you have to sweeten coffee or tea, I strongly suggest dumping the artificial sweeteners and instead using honey or a little regular table sugar. Skip the soda as much as possible. Water is best!

Aspartame is also known as Equal. It is found in beverages like sodas and flavored waters as well as chewing gum and light or sugar-free dairy products, ice creams, Popsicles, and other desserts. Aspartame is linked to birth defects, depression, epilepsy, multiple sclerosis, Alzheimer's disease, headaches, and neurological disorders. There have also been links found between aspartame and cancer. A European study published in the journal *Environmental Health Perspectives* found that low doses of aspartame resulted in lymphoma and leukemia cancers—in female rats only, interestingly.[52] The study stated that because testing of carcinogenicity in rodents, particularly rats and mice, provides a "consistent predictor of human cancer risk," more studies should be done on exposure levels, especially to shield children from any harmful exposure. While other studies claim that there is no link between cancer and aspartame, again, I like to be cautious and not wait until scientists all agree. The fact that aspartame is broken down and converted into formaldehyde (a known cancer causer) during digestion is reason enough for me to stay away.[53]

Sucralose is now the number one artificial sweetener on the market; you probably know it as Splenda and are likely familiar with its tagline: "Made from sugar, so it tastes like sugar." It is more accurate to say that it is *processed* into a chlorinated sugar, then mixed with dextrose and maltodextrin, which are made from corn. It's mistakenly believed to be a natural sugar due to the marketing that it is a derivative of sugar. In 2016, the Center for Science in the Public Interest, an American food and health watchdog group, downgraded sucralose's status from "caution" to "avoid" after the Ramazzini Institute, an independent laboratory based in Italy, found that the chemical caused leukemia and related blood cancers in male mice.[54] A study at Duke University also found that average to high consumption of Splenda reduced beneficial bacteria in the intestines of baby rats by as much as 50 percent. Beneficial bacteria help normalize weight and support immune function, among other things.[55] Sucralose is also thought to be a potential migraine trigger and has been linked to leukemia and other cancers in mice.[56] And beware of baking with it: when heated (especially at temperatures over 246°F/120°C), sucralose may form chlorinated organic compounds, such as chloropropanols, which are potentially toxic.[57] Instead, use one of the safer sweetener listed in this book.

Acesulfame potassium (or acesulfame K) is two hundred times sweeter than table sugar. The clear problem with this one is it contains the carcinogen methylene chloride. Long-term exposure to methylene chloride can cause headaches, depression, nausea, mental confusion, liver effects, kidney effects, visual disturbances, and cancer in humans.[58] However, the FDA has not called for further testing of it at this time, because they claim that previous testing on acesulfame potassium conducted in the 1970s indicated that it is safe.[59] However, researchers are calling for more studies due to concerns about the lack of long-term studies.

Saccharin (also known as Sweet'N Low) is two hundred to seven hundred times sweeter than regular sugar. Saccharin has a bitter aftertaste, so it's usually combined with other artificial sweeteners such as aspartame. It's found in carbonated drinks, jellies, and even medicines, mouthwash, and toothpaste. It came under fire in the 1970s when it was linked to bladder cancer in rats, but warnings were later retracted, although many scientists still believe there is a risk.[60] Animal studies showed rats given saccharin gained weight. Research has also shown that it may disturb gut flora, which—as we've discussed before—can lead to a whole host of health issues such as obesity, metabolic disorders, diabetes, inflammatory bowel disease, and cancer.

7. BHA and BHT

Butylated hydroxyanisole (BHA) and butylated hydroxytoluene (BHT) are antioxidant preservatives used in food. They are closely related synthetic antioxidant preservatives made from petroleum or coal tar and are commonly used in cosmetics as well as food. If you're not already a little bit freaked out by the words *coal tar*, you will be by the definition in the next sentence. Coal tar is a viscous, black liquid containing numerous organic compounds obtained by the destructive distillation of coal and is used as a roofing, waterproofing, and insulating compound. It is also a raw material for many dyes, drugs, and paints.

You will find BHA and BHT in artificial food colorings, cereals, snack foods, ice cream pies and cakes, processed meats, gum, and even beer. They're also sprayed into the lining of food packages to preserve freshness. You may see it on the label as "BHT added to packaging for freshness." The National Institutes of Health has said that BHA is "reasonably anticipated to be a human carcinogen."[61] It has also been found to interfere with hormone function, and in lab tests, long-term exposure to high doses of BHT caused liver, thyroid, and kidney problems in mice and rats.[62]

8. Benzoate preservatives

Usually on the labels of foods containing benzoate preservatives, you will see either sodium benzoate or potassium benzoate. Both are commonly found in beverages, especially soft drinks and flavored water. They can also be found in products like soy sauce, pickles, pepper rings, and tomato sauce. You might remember that I mentioned benzoate preservatives early on in the opening of this book, because it is one of the ingredients that I first eliminated myself. Because of Eric's attention issues, I looked into food ingredients that may exacerbate symptoms of ADHD, and benzoate preservatives were one of the first ones that I found. A 2007 British study published in the *Lancet* found a link between sodium benzoates and increased hyperactivity in children.[63] The researchers examined three hundred children in two different age groups: three-year-olds and eight- and nine-year-olds. Over three one-week periods, the children were randomly assigned to consume one of three fruit drinks daily. The first drink contained the amount of dye and sodium benzoate typically found in a British child's diet. The second drink had lower concentrations of the additives. Finally, the third drink was additive-free. All the children spent a week drinking each of the three mixtures, which looked and tasted alike. During each weeklong period, teachers and parents, who did not know which drinks the kids were getting, used a variety of evaluation and behavior tools to test their attention spans. Both of the additive-laden mixtures significantly affected the older kids, and the three-year-olds were affected by the mixture that was most potent and comparable to what a child is exposed to in their regular diet. As they evaluated the children, the teachers and parents noticed qualities like restlessness, concentration issues, and fidgeting as well as talking or interrupting too much among the kids who received the drinks with the additives. The results prompted lead researcher of the study, Jim Stevenson, to state that while the effects were not enough to cause a diagnosable case of ADHD, "the adverse effects could affect the child's ability to benefit from the experience of school."[64] The results of this study prompted Britain's food standards agency to issue an immediate advisory for parents to limit their children's intake of additives if they notice an effect on behavior.

There's also a cancer connection with benzoates. When combined with vitamin C in beverages—such as some soft drinks, fruit juices, and even some flavored water—benzoates can combine to form benzene, which is a known human carcinogen. While the FDA states that most of the beverages tested (which have low or very low levels of benzene) do not pose a safety concern, other studies state that more research is needed to understand the effects of long-term consumption of low levels of benzene.[65] Another study in 2011 on cultured human cells found that sodium benzoates significantly increased damage to DNA. These results indicated that sodium benzoate is "clastogenic, mutagenic, and cytotoxic to human lymphocytes in vitro."[66] This means that sodium benzoate can damage, break, or change DNA and that it is toxic to cells in the body, which can result in cell mutation and cancer.

What concerns me about sodium benzoate and potassium benzoate is the potential for multiple exposures over the course of a day from a variety of sources. I would rather err on the side of caution and just avoid them. If you decide to do the same, check items such as personal care products too. Sodium benzoate can be found in a lot of shampoos, mouthwash, and toothpaste. Look out for products with any of these ingredients listed on the label: sodium benzoate, potassium benzoate, or benzoic acid. Sometimes you'll also see it listed as E211, which is sodium benzoate, or E212, which is potassium benzoate.

9. Artificial colors

Artificial colors are petroleum-based dyes that make foods and beverages like candy, cereal, soda, and Popsicles more fun and colorful. They're used in many other processed goods to give color, such as chips, crackers, juices, pickles, ice cream, salad dressings—and even toothpaste, mouthwash, medicines, pills, and cough syrups. While they brighten foods and help give more uniform color, they offer no nutritional value, and may do more harm than good.

Although there are nine of these certified synthetic dyes approved use in the United States, Red No. 40, Yellow No. 5, and Yellow No. 6 account for the 90 percent used in foods (they may also be listed without the number sign, as in Red 40). These three colorings also contain benzidine, a known human and animal carcinogen, meaning this substance is known to cause cancer in humans and animals.[67]

Hypersensitivity is another problem with artificial food dyes. In addition to Red No. 40, the dyes Yellow No. 5, Yellow No. 6, Blue No. 1, and Red No. 4 (also called carmine) can cause allergic reactions, ranging from hives and itchy skin to facial swelling and flushing.[68] Reports of anaphylactic shock have also been reported with carmine.[69]

And remember the Southampton study in the previous section about benzoate preservatives and food colorings contributing to hyperactivity? That's another concern with artificial food colorings. In fact, a study published in the journal *Neurotherapeutics* states that artificial colors "are not a major cause of ADHD per se, but seem to affect children *regardless of whether or not* they have ADHD."[70]

Many of the foods in Europe have different formulations than they do here in the United States, and some of these food colorings have either been removed there or they must carry a warning label, such as "this product may have adverse effect on activity and attention in children."[71] Some colorings—such as turmeric, red beets, beta carotene, and saffron—are more natural and haven't been found to lead to hyperactive effects, so these would be a better option.

We're likely getting multiple exposures to these colorings several times a day, in our foods, beverages, toothpastes, cosmetics, and supplements. And many foods and beverages have multiple food colorings just in one product! To avoid artificial dyes, beware foods and beverages that list colors followed by a number on the ingredient label (such as Yellow #5), and eat and cook with whole foods as much as possible, limiting packaged foods.

10. GMOs

The research around genetically modified organisms (GMOs) has mixed results. GMOs are created when genes are taken from one species, such as a bacteria or virus, and are then placed into the DNA of other species, such as soybeans and corn plants.[72] After GMOs were introduced into the United States a few decades ago, some people began to report toxic effects from consuming them. One particular advocacy group, the Institute for Responsible Technology (IRT), reported that after feeding rats a diet that contained a genetically modified potato, nearly every organ in the rats' bodies were negatively affected after only a few days.[73] Many scientists across the world have sought to find out whether the IRT was right—if the process of genetically modifying food can cause toxicity. Hundreds of studies have been conducted to ascertain whether or not GMOs are a threat to human health. According to a 2015 report by a researcher at Harvard University, "knowing who to trust and what to believe regarding this topic is an ongoing battle."[74] But according to that report, major health groups, like the American Medical Association and the World Health Organization, have determined that there is no evidence suggesting that GMOs cause organ toxicity or adverse health effects.

The primary concern now about the health effects of GMOs is whether they may cause health problems for future generations. While scientists and consumers may continue to argue about whether or not GMOs are safe long term, I recommend clients avoid them to err on the side of caution. The way I suggest doing that is by eating organic foods as much as possible and buying products with the non-GMO label.

Now what? How do I eat *anything*?

OK, that was a lot to digest, I know. But remember, even just cutting out *one* of the ingredients in this chapter will make a difference in your health. You don't need to ditch all of them right away, and as always, I will remind you to stay focused on what's most important for *your* family. Remember when I asked you to define why you are choosing to go slightly greener? We're going to use your answer right now to figure out how you can improve what you're eating.

What's the top priority for your family right now?

A. Minimizing exposure

B. Losing weight

C. Alleviating symptoms

D. Throw it all at me, Tonya. I'm an overachiever!

If you answered A, concentrate on buying organic.

If you answered B, ditch the artificial sweeteners, sugary packaged foods, and MSG.

If you answered C, avoid MSG, artificial colors, and artificial sweeteners.

And if you answered D, chill, but seriously, prioritize organic foods, minimize processed and packaged products when you can, and read ingredient lists on the prepared stuff you buy. Easy-peasy.

Ingredients to Avoid in Food

INGREDIENT	FOUND IN	HEALTH EFFECTS
Natural flavors	Coffee creamer, oatmeal, fruit snacks, cereals, spices, beverages, soups, dairy products	• May hide ingredients such as MSG and gluten • Considered to be a proprietary formula, so individual ingredients are not required to be listed
Artificial flavors	Candy, chips, crackers, salad dressings, ice cream, cereal, fruit juices, flavored yogurt, toothpaste, and medicines	• Considered to be a proprietary formula so individual ingredients are not required to be listed • Made up of chemicals that can include preservatives, solvents, and other additives
High fructose corn syrup	Many processed foods, such as crackers, cookies, condiments, cereals, chips, jelly, and some vitamins	• Linked to diabetes, obesity, and metabolic disorder • Also linked to cancer and accelerated aging • GMO and possible mercury contamination
Monosodium glutamate	Most processed foods, such as chips, salad dressings, canned soups, sauces, flavored crackers, and in spices and flavorings (such as some taco seasonings and Accent flavor enhancer)	• Hides in over forty different ingredients • May excite neurons (nerve cells) to the point of cell death • May affect the development of the nervous system
Carrageenan	Dairy products such as ice cream, heavy whipping cream, ice cream, cottage cheese, and yogurt	• Linked to colitis and colon cancer • May contribute to weight gain • Interferes with beneficial flora in GI tract

INGREDIENT	FOUND IN	HEALTH EFFECTS
Artificial sweeteners	Sugar-free and diet foods and beverages, such as diet soda, sugar-free jelly, sugar-free Jell-O, flavored water, and Pedialyte. Includes brand names Splenda, Sweet'N Low, and Equal	· Linked to birth defects · May alter gut flora · Linked to neurological disorders, such as Alzheimer's and multiple sclerosis
Bisphenol A (BPA)	Plastics (such as plastic water bottles); also linings of most canned goods	· Linked to diabetes, heart disease, breast cancer, and toxicity to female reproductive system · Acts as a hormone disruptor
BHA and BHT	Snack foods, cereal, processed meats, gum, beer, and lining of food packages (will usually see "BHT added for freshness" on label)	· May be cancer causing · Sleep and behavior issues · Interferes with hormone function and may mimic estrogen
Benzoates	Foods and beverages such as soda, fruit juice, pickles, soy sauce, tomato sauce, and even in flavored water	· Linked to hyperactivity in children · Can form benzene (a known cancer causer) when combined with vitamin C
Artificial colors	Cereals, medicines, candy, toothpaste, Popsicles, frosting, canned vegetables, and ice cream	· Linked to hyperactivity · Some contain benzidine, a known cancer causer
GMOs	Many conventionally grown foods such as apples, sugar beets, canola, and corn	· Linked to infertility, immune issues, organ damage, accelerated aging, GI and organ problems, and problems with insulin regulation

6

Safe Water, Food Storage, and the Kitchen Cleanout

Now that we have covered what's in our food, it's time to turn our attention to how we cook and store it as well as how we wash it down. Then we will tackle the final and most fun part—the slightly greener kitchen cleanout! This is a final sweep to integrate all the things we've learned about slightly greener eating. Bonus: you will get an added benefit of a decluttering happiness boost.

Think about what you eat or drink on a typical day. Chances are good it involves one common element. See if you can guess it. You might start by microwaving yesterday's leftover oatmeal in a Tupperware container. Your morning routine might include coffee made from a Keurig pod, poured into a plastic tumbler for the morning commute. Lunch? A salad to go in a plastic container and plastic bag with a bottle of water. Are you recognizing a common ingredient? Plastic, plastic, plastic!

If you feel like it's everywhere, you're right. Plastic is used to heat, line, contain, serve, and store our food. But there's mounting evidence that all the plastic we're exposed to in our food and beverages can have repercussions on our health. My clients who have just learned about all the toxins *in* their food, now faced with the dangers of ubiquitous plastic all *around* it, start to panic. This is when I tend to see hands flailing in the air: "I can't do it!" But don't freak out. You *don't* have to try to eliminate all the plastic in your life.

By the time you finish reading this chapter, you will have a handful of practical food storage containers, an overview of how to shop for safe cookware, and safe drinking water tips. Just start with *one* change and build from there. First tip? Start with your plastic storage containers. If your kitchen is like most families', it's filled with plastic, especially if you have kids. My guess is that your cabinets are filled with plastic cups, plates, and everyone's favorite: Tupperware. But these familiar products can also cause us harm. The next time you go shopping or see an online sale, replace a few of your plastic containers with glass options, starting with just a couple of your most-used containers and occasionally replacing the rest as needed. There's the 80/20 rule in action right there—you probably use those few containers about 80 percent of the time, and now they are safer.

The problem with BPA

Bisphenol A (BPA) is an industrial chemical used to make polycarbonate, which is a hard, clear plastic.[1] It's used in many consumer products, but it's also added to the epoxy linings of many canned foods, like canned tomatoes and canned soups, so that the food doesn't touch the metal directly. The problem is that BPA works as an endocrine disruptor. BPA is linked to toxicity of the female reproductive system, which means that sexual function and fertility may be negatively impacted, as well as diabetes, heart disease, breast cancer, and even infertility.[2] A study conducted by researchers in the Department of Obstetrics, Gynecology, and Reproductive Sciences and the Department of Neurobiology at Yale found that low doses of BPA exposure impaired brain function and may lead to learning disabilities.[3]

Another challenge? There is *a lot* of BPA in our environment; over six billion pounds of BPA are produced each year.[4] It's found in plastic bottles, water bottles, canned foods, plastic food containers, and thermal paper receipts from stores, banks, and gas stations, even dental sealants put on kids' teeth! But if you live in California, there's some good news. In 2015, California added BPA to the list of chemicals known to cause harm to women's reproductive health, which means that products containing BPA now come with a warning label when sold in stores in California.

HOW TO AVOID BPA

→ Avoid canned food and drinks as much as possible.

→ Buy BPA-free canned foods.

→ Avoid plastic bottles and use glass or stainless steel instead.

→ Do not microwave plastic or put it through the dishwasher (heat can leech the plastic chemicals into food and drinks).

→ Ask for emailed store receipts or just say no if the receipt isn't needed.

→ If using plastic, look for recycle codes 1, 2, 4, or 5 (found on the bottom of most plastic bottles and containers with a number and arrows). AVOID recycle codes 3, 6, and 7. The American Academy of Pediatrics has previously noted that the recycling codes 3, 6, and 7 indicate the presence of phthalates, styrene, and bisphenols, in that order.

FUN FACT

Many receipts are now printed on thermal paper, which is coated with BPA or its close relative BPS. Research has also found that using hand sanitizer before touching your receipt may increase absorption of BPA into the skin by up to 185 times as opposed to when hands were dry.[5] Eating something greasy like French fries or even wearing hand lotion when touching the receipt can do the same. So I suggest asking for an email receipt as often as possible.

In 2018, the American Academy of Pediatrics sounded the alarm and called for urgent reform to the FDA regulatory process that reviews food additives. BPA's estrogen-like qualities can potentially bring about early puberty, which can lead to decreased fertility, increased weight gain, and may negatively alter important body systems, such as the nervous, immune, and cardiovascular systems.[6] In response to mounting pressure and advocacy from pediatricians, parents, and concerned citizens since 2012, BPA is no longer used in infant formula cans, baby bottles, or sippy cups. This is great news!

There has also been some research that links BPA to hyperactivity. A study published in *Environmental Research* states that prenatal and child-hood exposure to BPA have been linked to anxiety, depression, hyper-activity, and behavior issues in children.[7] The Yale School of Medicine found that low doses of BPA can negatively affect brain function, which can lead to learning disabilities and neurodevelopmental issues.[8] But one of the bigger problems is that the substitutes used for BPA have not been proven to be any safer. So even though a product may say it's BPA-free, if it's made of plastic, I still recommend avoiding it.

Don't trust BPA-free

BPA-free products have grown in popularity recently, but the reality is that they are made with chemicals that carry similar risks to BPA. In BPA-free products, the BPA is typically substituted with another bisphenol compound such as BPS or BPF, but studies have found that BPS and BPF are similar chemicals with similar health effects to BPA.

A study conducted at the University of Cincinnati found that exposing rats to BPS showed disruptive heart rhythms.[9] Another study from the New York University School of Medicine found a link between BPS and weight gain.[10] BPS treatment and possibly expo-sure resulted in gene signatures that suggest effects on metabolism, adiposity (which is when excessive abdominal fat builds up around the stomach), and insulin sensitivity (which is related to diabetes). Research from the University of Massachusetts at Amherst also found that BPS alters brain development and behavior.[11] In a study on zebrafish, exposure to both BPA and BPS during what is the equiv-alent of the second trimester for a developing human fetus altered the rate of neuron development in the hypothalamus.[12] Low levels of exposure to BPA resulted in a 180 percent increase in the neurons in the hypothalamus, while low levels of exposure to BPS resulted in a 240 percent increase. In layman's terms, the fish exposed to these chemicals showed significant signs of hyperactivity as adults due to the increase in neuron production during gestation.

The takeaway: use glass.

No plastics in the kitchen

It's not too hard to avoid BPA, because there *are* safer solutions. Here's the simple rule I follow: **no plastics in the kitchen**. I don't use plastic, and I don't let the kids do so either. Our kitchen cabinets are filled with all glass, and I use glass or wood products for measuring spoons and cooking utensils. Truth be told: my hubby has a couple of plastic cups he uses outside, but he's the only one in our family who uses them. (Listen, I can't control him all the time, but I've got him about 80 percent trained! See! The 80/20 rule is useful for lots of things— even spouses. Try it!)

Lifefactory, S'well, and Klean Kanteen all make stainless steel or glass reusable water bottles that are BPA-free. They have great colors and design and are easy for either you or your kids to carry.

The EWG also has a great section on BPA-free foods. When you go to the site, it will give you the names of brands that don't contain BPA.

How to choose safer cookware

Now that you've gotten a handle on the plastic in your food storage—or at least selected a safer option for your most-used food storage containers—it's time to examine your cookware. When it comes to choosing safe cookware, there are a lot of options out there. But first, I don't think there's necessarily a perfect pan out there. There are some that I believe are less safe than others and shouldn't be used, as you'll see, but it sometimes depends on what you're cooking, how long you're cooking it for, and whether or not it's damaged. While I use ceramic cookware a lot of the time, I do love to break out my cast iron for certain meals!

While nonstick pans tend to be a consumer favorite because they are so easy to clean up after cooking, unfortunately, they're not the safest choice.

Bummer, I know.

We may not think of cookware as a potential health threat, but just as with BPA in our canned foods and in Tupperware, the chemicals from cookware can also get into our bodies. Harmful chemical exposure can occur as pots and pans heat up, and we can become exposed to toxins when they leach into the food during cooking or when we inhale the fumes. Chemicals can also leach into food if the cookware is scratched. But with so many different cookware brands, in addition to an overwhelming amount of information available, how do we know which pots and pans to use?

First, I stay away from Teflon or nonstick cookware, which is the standard you tend to see in kitchens everywhere, as nonstick cookware is incredibly popular! In 2019, U.S. retail sales of nonstick cookware amounted to approximately $1.47 billion.[13] That's *a lot* of nonstick frying pans! Teflon is a synthetic chemical made up of carbon and fluorine atoms and was first created in the 1930s to create a desirable nonstick and nonreactive surface.[14] You've probably used a nonstick pan covered in Teflon for the same reasons I have: the pancakes flip easily, the omelets lift up perfectly, and there's practically no mess left over when the meal is ready.

But for the last decade, nonstick cookware has been under investigation due to safety concerns. The reason? Teflon can release toxic fumes when it gets hot. There has long been concern over a chemical called perfluorooctanoic acid, which was long used in the nonstick coating but has not been in use since 2013. Today, a chemical called *polytetrafluoroethylene* is used on nonstick pans instead. But according to tests commissioned by the EWG, in as little as two minutes on the stovetop, "cookware coated with Teflon and other nonstick surfaces can exceed temperatures at which the coating breaks apart and emits toxic particles and gases linked to hundreds, perhaps thousands, of pet bird deaths and an unknown number of human illnesses each year."[15] *Yikes.* So when you preheat a pan or turn a burner on high heat, it's possible that harmful toxins are emitted into the air. This is a condition known as *Teflon toxicosis*, which can cause a bird's lungs to hemorrhage and fill with fluid, leaving the bird to die of suffocation. All for speedy cleanup after scrambling eggs? No thank you. Even if you do keep the temperature lower and at a "safe" level, the chemicals can still leach over time due to wear and tear or if the pans gets damaged or scratched.

I also steer clear of aluminum cookware, as studies have demonstrated that aluminum from cookware can leach into foods, and research has shown that excess aluminum in the body is linked to Alzheimer's disease and other neurodegenerative diseases.[16]

Cast iron cookware is a popular option, and it has a lot of benefits. It's durable and stays hot, and its seasoning makes it naturally nonstick. It's a great option for cooking eggs, baking, sautéing veggies, searing meat, or making a pancake breakfast. (And who doesn't love a warm, gooey chocolate chip cookie baked in a skillet?)

Another positive aspect of cooking with cast iron is that small amounts of iron can leach into food when heated. If you need to add a little more iron to your diet, that's great. But for some people with rare conditions, such as the genetic condition of iron overload (hemochromatosis), it's not recommended.[17] It seems like cooking with cast iron might not necessarily be a significant source of iron, but in fact, doing so can greatly increase the amount of iron absorbed into the food. According to a study published in the *Journal of the American Dietetic Association*, "90 percent of foods tested contained *significantly* more iron when cooked in iron utensils than when cooked in non-iron utensils."[18] Researchers in this study found that factors such as acidity and cooking time increased the absorption of iron into the food. Avoid cooking foods that are acidic, such as lemon juice and tomato sauce, in your cast iron cookware. Doing so can break down the seasoning and can leach more iron into food, also giving it a metallic taste. Avoiding cooking foods that require a longer cooking time in cast iron can also cut down on the amount of iron absorbed into the food.

Caring for cast iron cookware is simple as long as you follow a few basic tips. While these tips are pretty universal for cast iron care, I always recommend checking your specific brand's care instructions just to be sure. One of the most important things is to avoid scrubbing cast iron with anything abrasive, such as steel wool. This can remove the seasoning, allowing more iron to leach into foods and also leaving a metallic taste behind. Lodge Cast Iron cookware's website recommends using a sponge and warm water to gently scrape off foods and then completely dry. While some of my clients say they've heard that soap is not recommended, Lodge states that a small amount of soap is just fine if needed. If there is stuck-on residue, you can use a chain-mail sponge or a pan scraper for those heavy-duty jobs. Chain-mail sponges offer just enough texture without being too abrasive, but they're not recommended for everyday use. Steel wool or metal scrubbers are only recommended when removing rust before reseasoning the cookware.[19]

CAST IRON COOKWARE TIPS

→ Preheat cast iron for best results.

→ Don't cook acidic items, such as lemon juice or tomato sauce.

→ Don't store foods in cast iron. Remove as soon as finished cooking.

→ Don't scrub with steel wool or anything abrasive.

→ Use a sponge and water to clean (a small amount of soap is fine, if needed).

→ Use a chain-mail sponge for heavy residue.

→ Dry completely after washing. Don't soak cast iron, because it can rust.

Stainless steel sounds good for preparing meals right? Well, there are some leaching concerns with stainless steel cookware too. The reason is that stainless steel also contains the metals nickel and chromium in its composition.[20] In certain instances, the nickel can leach into the food, particularly with high acidity foods like tomatoes, which is a concern for some people who—like me—have a nickel sensitivity.[21] You also shouldn't use stainless steel when damaged or scratched, as that can cause nickel exposure as well. On the bottom of the cookware, you will see numbers. The first number is for chromium, followed by the nickel content. Ideally, look for 18/8 or 18/0, which have the lowest percentage of nickel possible.

For my own cooking, I use ceramic cookware a majority of the time. There are two different types of ceramic cookware: pure ceramic cookware and cookware that is covered with a ceramic-like coating. You want to look for the pure ceramic cookware. The ceramic-covered cookware is made with polymer materials that *look* like ceramic. Only with the pure ceramic option, there is less leaching of heavy metals, and you can be more certain that your food won't be tainted with chemicals during the cooking or heating process.

FOUR STEPS TO SAFE COOKWARE

1. Don't preheat pans without food or liquid in them.

2. Cook at a lower heat, especially if using nonstick pans.

3. Don't store foods in pans, as chemicals can leach into foods.

4. Replace cookware that has visible scratches or damage.

After you've tackled safer cookware in the kitchen (or at least replaced your most-used pots and pans), next I suggest paying attention to the water you drink.

Is my water safe?

The average human body is made of 60 percent water.[22] We have to consume it to live; the average person needs about five liters a day to survive. It's no surprise that drinking water is essential for good health, and the quality of the water is paramount. Most of us know that unfiltered tap water can be contaminated with harmful chemicals like chlorine, pesticides, heavy metals, and even hexavalent chromium. We've also seen headlines in the news about contaminated water, like in 2015 when dangerous levels of lead were detected in drinking water in Flint, Michigan. A study from the *Proceedings of the National Academy of Sciences* found that since 1982, 3–10 percent of U.S. water systems have violated the federal standards outlined by the Safe Drinking Water Act, affecting forty-five million people.[23] Tap water is safe in the large majority of cases, but it *can* be unsafe, so it's important to know what's in the water we drink.

Bottled water is a tempting option for some consumers. In addition to the added convenience of a grab-and-go bottle of water, many people feel like it is a healthier, safer option and worth the added cost. But here is one of the biggest misconceptions I bust for my clients: *bottled water isn't necessarily a better option*. In fact, according to the Mayo Clinic, the safety of tap water is almost always comparable to bottled water.[24] Tap water is regulated by the EPA and is often tested for organisms like cryptosporidium. It's also disinfected and filtered to remove chemicals or pathogens. The FDA is responsible for ensuring the safety (and label accuracy) of bottled water sold in the United States. The key distinction here is that city water may be tested for bacteria and organic compounds one hundred or more times a month, whereas a bottled water plant may be required to test only once a week. Additionally, a recent Consumer Reports investigation found that information on bottled water can be hard to find. Its oversight is often inconsistent, and—like tap water—it can be contaminated.[25]

The takeaway here: tap water, while not 100 percent perfect, is more closely regulated.

Before you run out to buy a chemistry set and start testing your own water every night, know there's a simple solution.

Drink filtered tap water

Because it is more closely regulated, I recommend that you drink tap water and use a filtering device inside your home. There are simple steps you can take to find out if the tap water in your neighborhood is safe. First, call your water company and ask for an annual water quality report, also called a consumer confidence report. I also suggest you go to the EWG's Tap Water Database (ewg.org/tapwater) and type in your zip code to learn about the quality of the water you drink.[26] If you learn that your water *isn't* healthy, then I recommend getting a filter. EWG's Tap Water database also has a great database of filters, where you can enter your zip code and receive filter recommendations in response to the specific qualities of your water.[27]

You might be saying, "But I love my bottled water!" I know many of us have been led to believe that bottled water is cleaner, safer, and better. But remember what I said about food labels and how they trick consumers with works like *natural?* The next time you look at the label on a bottle of water, take a discerning look at the mouth-watering geysers and springs overflowing with crystal-clear water.

Once again, those labels are mostly marketing ploys, not reality.

The problem with bottled water

A recent report by a nonprofit organization called Food & Water Watch stated that 64 percent of bottled water comes from the tap.[28] Back in 1999, the Natural Resources Defense Council completed a four-year study of the bottled water industry and stated "that there is no assurance that bottled water is cleaner or safer than tap. In fact, an estimated 25 percent or more of bottled water is really just tap water in a bottle— sometimes further treated, sometimes not."[29] A Consumer Reports investigation also made the news recently when it revealed that several popular bottled water brands sold water with elevated levels of arsenic—a heavy metal that can negatively impact child development— at or above a threshold research suggests is potentially dangerous to drink over an extended period of time.[30] Drinking one bottle of water containing arsenic over the suggested limit probably isn't harmful, but long-term consumption *is* linked to lower IQ and may cause certain cancers and other health problems like cardiovascular disease.[31]

Not convinced yet? Well, it's not just arsenic that causes problems in bottled water. There's also the concern of chemicals leaching into the water from plastic water bottles. Chemicals such as BPA and phthalates have been found in water stored in plastic water bottles for as little as ten weeks.[32] These chemicals are linked to hormone disruption as well as lower IQ and behavior issues in children, among other health effects. Chemical leaching from hard plastic can occur faster—and in greater amounts—when the plastic is exposed to heat. The most common example is leaving a water bottle, or any plastic container, in a hot car. It doesn't help to then stick the bottle in the refrigerator—the chemicals have already leached into the water. Something else to consider is the heat bottled water can be exposed to *before* we purchase it. What if the truck that shipped the water bottles was hot? Or what if the water bottles were stored in a hot room at any point along the distribution channel? Even if the water that originally went into that plastic bottle was perfectly safe, if it's heated or stored in plastic too long, there's a risk that chemical agents or phthalates can leach into the water itself.

And then there's the issue of what our massive plastic addiction is doing to our planet. While it's beyond the scope of this book to go into detailed environmental analysis, I'd like to add a few key points about the sheer volume of plastic in our world today and the challenges it poses. Bottled water causes a *huge* carbon footprint. Scientists have found that human beings have produced more than eight billion tons of plastic, largely since the 1950s.[33] This is the equivalent to the weight of a billion elephants and will last for hundreds, if not thousands, of years. Less than 10 percent of it has been recycled. The *Guardian* found that there are a million plastic bottles purchased every minute.[34] That's twenty thousand bottles a second. These plastics pile up in landfills, and slowly, over time, they break down into microplastics, which are tiny particles of plastic. These microplastics seep into soil, rivers, lakes, and oceans, eventually landing in—and contaminating—our food and water supply. Research on the health effects of microplastics is still new, so it's hard to say what the effect of all *that* plastic is on humans. And if you haven't yet been convinced to ditch plastic water bottles, there's the cost. According to *Business Insider*, bottled water costs two thousand times more than tap.[35]

It's clear: we all need to do our part to put less plastic into the world, starting with the kitchen. Rather than quit because you feel defeated, start small: no plastic water bottles.

IF YOU HAVE TO PURCHASE BOTTLED WATER

→ Choose your bottled water brands carefully!

→ Go on the company website to see if they publish test results on the safety of their water.

→ Check the label and the cap. If it says "from a municipal source" or "from a community water system," that bottle is filled with tap water, not water from a natural spring!

THREE EASY TIPS FOR SAFE WATER

1. **Drink filtered tap water.** There are simple filters you can use, such as Brita or Pur, that you fill with water and keep in the fridge. (In this instance, the plastic is OK to use, because it's not being heated

or frozen.) You can also use activated charcoal sticks, which work
well and typically last longer than the pitchers. Activated charcoal
can remove contaminants such as heavy metals and chlorine.

2. **Find the best filter for your water.** The EWG has a great Tap Water
Database. Just type in your zip code, and it will tell you what's in
your water and the best filter for it.

3. **Use glass or stainless-steel water bottles.** Take water on the go
in glass or stainless-steel bottles instead of using bottled water
or plastic reusable water bottles. A couple of my favorite reusable
water bottles are S'well, Klean Kanteen, and Lifefactory.

If you're having plastic anxiety right now, I don't blame you. It comes down to a problem of speed. Innovation (new plastics, chemicals, and products) happens at the speed of light. Regulation (Is it safe? Are we sure? How much is too much? What should the laws be?) moves more like a snail. According to a study in the *Journal of Environmental Science and Technology*, there are widespread toxicity issues in everyday plastics.[36] Scientists say we just don't know enough about the slew of chemicals in our everyday plastic products. This study examined thirty-four everyday plastic products made from eight different types of plastic and found that 74 percent of the products were toxic in some way. We tend to think of plastic as a single ingredient, but it is made from mixtures of thousands of chemicals, many of which may have effects on the human body that are currently unknown.

Simple kitchen and pantry cleanout

Now that we've covered our food, how we store it, and how we wash it down, it's time to tackle a full kitchen cleanout. I've come up with an easy method to transform what's in your kitchen, without overwhelming feelings or the guilt that inevitably comes when you realize you want to throw out half your pantry. This method allows you to change the foods you eat over time, which prevents the food fights that happen when your teenage daughter realizes you're tossing her beloved Kraft Macaroni & Cheese.

Step 1: Prepare

Decide whether you're going to clear out your whole pantry/kitchen or just one shelf/area/storage space. Clear a counter or table to put everything on. Pull everything out and sort the items into **four** categories:

- Items you use nearly every day
- Items you use less frequently
- Unopened, unexpired products that can be donated to a food pantry
- Expired items to throw away

Clean the empty shelves. A quick vacuum will make your life so much easier. Follow that with a spray bottle mixture of vinegar and water. Good as new!

Step 2: Sort unopened and expired items

Place unopened items to donate into a bag, and throw away the expired items.

Step 3: Separate items by frequency of consumption

With the donated and expired foods gone, the two groups left are items you frequently use and those you use only on an occasional basis. Look at the foods your family consumes most often. These will be the ones you think about replacing first.

Step 4: Remove your deal breaker ingredients

These are the ingredients that you have decided to absolutely avoid. I recommend avoiding aspartame and other artificial sweeteners as an important place to start. A quick list of other ingredients that may be included in your deal breakers is below:

- MSG
- Carrageenan
- Artificial colors
- High fructose corn syrup
- BHA/BHT

- BPA (canned goods, plastic containers, water bottles)
- Natural & artificial flavors
- GMOs
- Benzoate preservatives

Step 5: Replace discarded items with a healthier version

Begin replacing those items you got rid of for ones that are free of your deal-breaker ingredients (you can do this just one or two items at a time).

When you're finished, do the same for your refrigerator, and remember to check your beverages too!

Remember, this is not about being perfect! You can definitely choose to toss these toxins and replace your food all at once, but you can also choose the one or two items you use the most and begin by just replacing those. If you do that every couple of weeks, you'll have a healthier pantry before you know it!

FOURTEEN SIMPLE TIPS FOR SLIGHTLY GREENER EATING ON A BUDGET!

1. **Replace just the two or three foods your family consumes the most** with a healthier version. For instance, if your child's favorite food is hot dogs, switch to a healthier brand.

2. **Eat/shop seasonally.** Seasonal foods don't have to travel as far, keeping their nutrients, and they will typically be cheaper. To find what is in season in your area, see the list of websites and apps in the Resources section.

3. **Only buy organic of the produce listed on the EWG's Dirty Dozen list.** These are the foods that are highest in pesticides.

4. **Buy your organic foods at warehouse and membership club stores.** Buying in bulk, especially in bulk bins of the foods you frequently eat, can save a lot of money in the long run.

5. **Check your store's policy on stacking coupons.** Download coupons from the store's website, and look online for coupons for that same product. Some stores will honor the double coupons.

6. **Shop the store's own organic brands.** Those brands have to adhere to the same organic requirements, but the product will be cheaper because you are not paying for labels and marketing. For example, Whole Foods has the 365 brand, and Target has Simply Balanced.

7. **Don't buy prewashed produce.** It can cost almost twice as much, plus you'll most likely rewash it anyway!

8. **Join a CSA.** A CSA (community supported agriculture) is typically a group whose members receive weekly shares of food from a certain farm (or group of farms) in their area. Although the cost may seem steep upfront (it is usually paid upfront), the breakdown is an average of only $12 to $18 per week.

9. **Plant your own garden if possible.** If you don't have an area in your backyard, do some research to see if garden community space is available.

10. **Decide on your deal-breaker ingredients.** For instance, if you want to avoid MSG, avoid all foods with that in it. If you decide organic dairy is important to you, then only buy that but maybe skimp in some other areas. Again, this is not about being perfect.

11. **Find the brands you like on social media** sites, such as Facebook, Instagram, and Twitter, and follow them. They will often post coupons for their followers.

12. **Google the company name plus "coupons"** and see if anything pops up (for example, google "Vermont Soap Organics + Coupons"). If nothing comes up, sign up for their newsletter list; many companies frequently email deals and coupons.

13. **Shop websites such as Vitacost and Amazon.** You'll get free shipping on Prime items if you are an Amazon Prime member, and Vitacost offers free shipping on orders over $49.

14. **Check out Thrive Market.** This is an online membership store that carries natural and organic products at wholesale prices, but be sure to check food and product labels carefully to find any ingredients that might be on your deal-breaker list.

Part III

Slightly Greener Cosmetics

7

Don't Be Fooled by Cosmetic Labels

If a cosmetic is being sold commercially, it has to be safe, right?

Wrong.

Companies that manufacture personal care products (like shampoos, lotions, perfumes, makeup, and even toothpaste) have appallingly little safety accountability. According to a 2019 *New York Times* article, "the FDA's oversight of the cosmetics industry remains astoundingly limited."[1] The article goes on to explain that the FDA "cannot require companies to submit safety data before they market a product, to adhere to basic manufacturing standards once they do, or even to register with the agency, things drug and medical device makers are mandated to do."

Feeling nervous about your morning beauty routine? It gets worse.

The article adds, "Companies don't even have to report

problems—or 'adverse events'—that consumers relay to them. And if regulators do hear of incidents, they cannot demand to be allowed to inspect a company's records; they can only check a facility for visible flaws, like mold."

What? Did I just read that right? Companies that create the creams and powders we slather all over ourselves don't have to follow standards, submit safety data, or even report it if someone gets ill from their product?

That's right.

It's shocking to learn how little regulation there is in the cosmetics industry. But before you slam down this book and decide you just can't take another sentence of this toxin stuff, take a deep breath. Remember why moms like me and concerned consumers like you are sounding the alarm and creating change. You don't have to toss all your beauty products all at once; you only need to follow the Slightly Greener Method. Here's why you should avoid dangerous chemicals in your beauty products *some of the time*: if you start now, your incremental changes will build. Years from now, you will have greatly reduced your toxic load—a very smart step for your health and for that of your family. I think one day we will look back on blindly buying cosmetics like we do now on people in the 1960s not wearing seat belts—it's risky.

Let's take a closer look at some upsetting flaws in our regulatory system. The FDA's website states that under the Federal Food, Drug, and Cosmetic Act, "the law *does not* require cosmetic products and ingredients, other than color additives, to have FDA approval before they go on the market."[2] Instead, that power lies with the Cosmetic Ingredient Review panel. It is *their* responsibility to test the safety of the chemicals used in makeup and personal care products, and they meet quarterly to review the safety of cosmetic ingredients. But there are several issues with the Cosmetic Ingredient Review panel itself. First, the panel has only tested 11 percent of ingredients that go into personal care products.[3] That means that *89 percent of what's in cosmetics has never been tested* individually, let alone for synergistic or cumulative effects.

The second major flaw with the Cosmetic Ingredient Review panel is that it is funded by the Personal Care Products Council, which is comprised of leaders from the very companies they seek to regulate. Their 2019 Year in Review publication clearly shows that their board members are employees and executives at companies like Estée Lauder, Rodan and Fields, Revlon, Colgate-Palmolive, and Unilever.[4] That means the only entity that checks on what goes into cosmetics (as well as bath and body products) is comprised of leaders at the very companies that make—and profit from!—those products. If that doesn't present a conflict of interest, I don't know what does.

Here's a striking comparison. The European Union has banned over thirteen hundred chemicals and cosmetics, while the United States has banned just eleven.[5] In 2004, the EWG investigated seventy-five hundred personal care products and found that 99.6 percent of them contain one or more ingredients that have never been tested for safety by the Cosmetics Ingredient Review panel. One-third of all products contain ingredients linked to cancer, 70 percent may be contaminated with harmful impurities, and 55 percent contained penetration enhancers.[6] Penetration enhancers allow more ingredients—whether they're toxic or not—to readily penetrate the skin and get into the bloodstream quickly. Some of the penetration enhancers found included known or probable human carcinogens.

Another shocking fact: cosmetic legislation in the United States hasn't been updated since 1938![7]

Companies and individuals that manufacture or market cosmetics *do* have a legal responsibility to ensure the safety of their product, so they are responsible for truth in what they say, but they are entirely self-regulated. As consumers, it's hard to know what actually goes into the makeup, lotion, and body wash we use every day. In this chapter as well as the next, I'll tell you exactly what to look for on labels so you are more educated about what you're buying and can make small changes to stay safer and healthier. I'll also share some easy tips on how to reduce your overall exposure to harmful ingredients.

SLIGHTLY GREENER SKIN AND BODY TIP

Do not fall for slick marketing on personal care labels. These terms do not mean the product is safe! You need to read ingredient labels.

→ Mom approved!

→ Dermatologist (or pediatrician) recommended!

→ Vegan

→ Eco-friendly

→ Nontoxic

→ Hypoallergenic

The problem with personal care products and kids

Because of the speed at which they develop, children are particularly vulnerable to the negative effects of harmful chemicals in personal care products. As you will see in the coming pages, there are several harmful chemicals that act as endocrine disruptors in shampoos, body washes, and toothpaste—even those marketed for babies or touted as safe according to "pediatricians." Research has also shown that babies are *ten times* more vulnerable to the chemicals in personal care products than adults are.[8] According to the Children's Environmental Health Center at the Icahn School of Medicine at Mount Sinai in New York City, endocrine disruptors are suspected of contributing to reproductive and developmental disorders, weight gain, learning problems, and immune system dysfunction.[9] As I've mentioned earlier, children today are experiencing increasing rates of many health problems, particularly obesity. According to Dr. David Ludwig, director of a childhood obesity program at a Boston hospital, kids today will enter adulthood heavier than they've been at any time in human history.[10] As we learned when we talked about BPA, research suggests that rapid weight gain during infancy or later childhood might be related to maternal or early-life exposure to endocrine disruptors. It's entirely possible that endocrine disruptors play a role in the obesity epidemic, as exposure to them in utero can alter regular cells into becoming fat cells even before birth, and those cells stay with you for life.

There are alarming changes happening in children's reproductive health too. About 15 percent of American girls are expected to start puberty at age seven.[11] The age at which girls enter puberty has been decreasing for the last several decades. At the turn of the twentieth century, the average American girl got her period at the age of sixteen or seventeen, but in the last thirty years, that age has dropped to about twelve. Boys are entering puberty earlier now too.[12] A study published in the journal *Human Reproduction* looked at chemicals commonly found in personal care products—like toothpaste and makeup—and found that the daughters of mothers with higher levels of those chemicals in their urine during pregnancy faced a greater risk of entering puberty earlier.[13] Puberty at an earlier age is linked with an increased risk of breast and ovarian cancer in girls, testicular cancer in boys, and mental illness in both.

A 2008 study by the EWG found elevated risk with endocrine disruptor exposure among teens too. Like early childhood, adolescence is a time of rapid development: the reproductive, immune, blood, and adrenal hormone systems are going through huge shifts and maturation, and there are also critical shifts happening in the brain. Emerging research shows that adolescent girls are particularly vulnerable to the negative effects of endocrine disruptors in ways that can impact their long-term physical and emotional health.[14] Twenty of the teens tested in that 2008 EWG report had an average of thirteen hormone-altering cosmetics chemicals in their bodies. That particular report collected data on teens' exposure to parabens for the first time. Parabens are another endocrine disruptor found in about 85 percent of personal care products, usually as a preservative to prevent the growth of bacteria.[15] The results indicated that young women are widely exposed to parabens, most likely because of the number of products they use. Two in particular (methylparaben and propylparaben) were detected in *every single girl tested*.

The power of small changes to your beauty routine

Consider my client Lauren, who always had dry skin. When she moved to Wyoming a few years ago with her husband and two children, her face felt chapped during the harsh winter months. As a middle school teacher, Lauren—like all working mothers—was super busy; she never gave much thought to the skin care she used. She had used the same face cleanser and moisturizer for years. The label said it was safe ("dermatologist recommended!"), and it had even won some beauty awards. She trusted the label and didn't have time to research skin care.

Lauren had just started thinking about toxicity when she contacted me. Together we went through her personal care products, and I told her about the most toxic chemicals commonly found in them. She stopped using her face cleanser after she learned it contained sodium lauryl sulfate (SLS), which is linked to eczema and allergies. Her previously trusted cleanser also contained "parfum," another word for fragrance, which has been connected to weight problems, hormone disruption, cancer, and brain health issues in addition to eczema and allergies. Often, my clients come to me with an annoying but minor health issue like skin irritation or allergies. These issues appear like a warning signal, as though the body is saying, *Stop putting this stuff on me.* I work with many people like Lauren who don't initially suspect that their health issue could stem from personal care products. They are shocked to find a connection.

Lauren *thought* she was making a good choice, but when she looked at the fine print on her cosmetic labels, she realized that ingredients labeled "safe" were *not.* Since she switched to a safer product containing none of the ingredients I recommend avoiding, Lauren has enjoyed beautifully moisturized skin, even in the harsh Wyoming winters. And thanks to that little warning message from her skin, she has also reduced her exposure to harsh chemicals linked to more severe health issues, like cancer and hormone disruption. "I had no idea what was hiding in there," Lauren told me after learning my methods for reading product labels. "But now," she added, "it's practically automatic."

THE WORST CHEMICALS IN PERSONAL CARE PRODUCTS, RANKED

1. Formaldehyde releasers: can cause cancer

2. Parabens: can cause hormone disruption and weight gain; important to avoid in pregnancy

3. Fragrance/Parfum: can cause cancer, brain health issues, weight issues, hormone disruption, eczema, and allergies; important to avoid in pregnancy

4. Phthalates: can cause weight issues, hormone disruption, eczema, and allergies; important to avoid in pregnancy

5. Ethanolamines (DEA, MEA, TEA): risk of nitrosamine contamination

6. 1,4-dioxane: a probable cancer causer

7. Triclosan: can cause hormone disruption; important to avoid in pregnancy

8. Sodium lauryl sulfate: can cause eczema, allergies, and skin irritation

9. Methylisothiazolinone: can cause brain health issues, eczema, and allergies

10. Mineral oil: can be contaminated with cancer causers

11. Carrageenan: can cause cancer and weight issues

So much makeup, so many chemicals

Using cosmetics to cleanse, protect, or improve the physical appearance of our human bodies is not a new phenomenon. In fact, human beings have been rubbing things on their bodies and slathering tinctures on their skin for thousands of years. It's believed that Cleopatra took milk baths to make her skin lighter. Our ancestors may not have injected Botox into their foreheads or undergone plastic surgery to tame saggy skin, but they *did* create personal care concoctions to sharpen their looks. Fun fact: in 2003, archaeologists uncovered what is believed to be the oldest face cream; it is thought to be made from starch and animal fat! We're not alone in wanting to eliminate fine lines and under-the-eye puffiness. Apparently, our ancient ancestors did too.

But today, the health concerns of toxins in cosmetics include cancer, hormone disruption, developmental and reproductive toxicity, and bioaccumulation.[16] When toxins from cosmetics build up in the body, they are usually stored in fat cells, and that is one of the ways these chemicals can add to weight gain, which we will focus on the next chapter.

Cleopatra also wasn't assaulted with advertisements, marketing campaigns, influencers on social media, TV, podcasts, radio, and bill-boards convincing her that her all her problems would melt away if she would just buy a twelve-dollar bottle of night cream. A statistical survey found that in 2018, the beauty sector spent $18.3 billion on advertising.[17] In the United States and in the world at large, beauty is *big* business.

Not only are ridiculous sums of money spent to convince us we need to buy beauty products, there are now approximately 12,500 *different* chemical ingredients approved for use in the manufacture of personal care products.[18] Think about that for a second—just trying to picture what a lab full of 12,500 different chemicals would look like is mind-blowing.

And all those advertising dollars work: we use a *whole heck of a lot* of personal care products. According to a 2017 Statista survey, the average adult uses twenty to twenty-five different beauty or personal care products each day.[19] During her daily application of creams, lotions, sprays, deodorant, makeup and hair care, the aver-age woman is exposed to 168 chemical ingredients.[20] Now ponder *that* for a minute. And the average person who uses personal care prod-ucts daily can absorb almost *five pounds* of chemicals into their body each year.[21] That means that in the average human lifetime, we've potentially absorbed around *four hundred pounds* of chemicals into our bodies.

What's actually in cosmetics, anyway?

Most of the personal care products we use are made up of water, preservatives, emulsifiers, moisturizers, colors, thickeners, and fragrances. And it's true that some of these ingredients are safe, but not all are. Fragrance and some preservatives land at the top of my "avoid" list, because based on the research, those are some of the most harmful chemicals. Preservatives in cosmetics, like in food, have an important job. They keep mold, bacteria, and fungi from growing in the product. Who wants to put on rancid lipstick? But before we dive into which ingredients to avoid, let's first talk a little bit more about how chemicals from personal care products can be absorbed into the body in the first place.

How chemicals enter our bodies

Remember, there are three main ways that any toxin can enter your body. The first is *inhalation*, breathing in gases, fumes, or particles through your nose or mouth. This is what happens with perfumes, aerosol sprays, mists, toners, and fumes from nail polish or nail polish remover. The second way is through *absorption*: chemicals enter the body through your skin or eyes from eye makeup, lotion, sunscreen, shampoo, body wash, skin care products, deodorant, etc. The third way is *ingestion*, which could include anything you swallow but also things that go into your mouth, like mouthwash, toothpaste, teeth whiteners, etc.

Skin

The skin is the body's largest organ, accounting for more than 10 percent of body mass. It has a number of important jobs, including but not limited to protecting our vulnerable insides from being exposed to the elements, preserving water, absorbing shock, giving us tactile sensation, and temperature control.[22]

Believe it or not, applying products and absorbing chemicals through the skin actually may be more harmful than eating them. Think about drugs that are applied to the skin for absorption into the body, like nicotine patches or birth control medication. One of the biggest reasons for concern about the ingredients in personal care products is that the skin has been found to be a method of absorption rather than a true barrier. Many chemicals, including these toxins, can absorb into our bodies through the skin and bioaccumulate. Warm water (a.k.a. heat!) can impact absorption of some chemicals, so as we're showering or bathing our kids, the water could be making the effects worse.

When you eat a food that contains a toxin or an unnatural chemical, it goes through a process with enzymes to help break it down, detoxify it, and flush it out of the body. For this process to work properly, you must be healthy and have the proper enzymes to break the chemicals down as well as mature and healthy detoxification pathways to remove toxins. However, when you're applying a product to the skin, the chemical can absorb directly into the bloodstream without any sort of filtering system. Eye makeup can be absorbed through the porous mucus membranes around the eyes. Things such as lotions, shaving creams, shampoos, conditioners, foundations, and sunscreens can all be absorbed through the skin.

If you're freaking out and getting ready to swear off beauty products all together, don't worry. Unless you're having any particular health issues, I want you to start with your toothpaste. That's it!

Start with toothpaste

It makes sense, right? Even though we don't swallow toothpaste and we only use it in small quantities, it goes directly into our mouths twice a day! I was really surprised to learn how many toothpastes contain toxic ingredients, even some of the so-called natural brands. The mouth is one of the most absorbent parts of the body, giving toxins a fast track to your bloodstream. Have you ever heard that during a heart attack or chest pain, patients are told to take nitroglycerin sublingually, meaning under the tongue, or to dissolve it between the tongue and the cheek? That's because that area in the mouth is full of capillaries (tiny blood vessels) that allow drugs to quickly absorb into the bloodstream. When that happens, chemicals bypass the digestive system and any detoxification that may have taken place there.

SLIGHTLY GREENER BATHROOM SHOPPING

When you're about to pick up a new toothpaste, soap, or cleanser, there are two particular things to look out for:

→ If a product has triclosan in it, leave it on the shelf.

→ Avoid buying anything labeled "antibacterial."

There are some other challenges with toothpaste too. It can contain triclosan, which is an antibacterial and antifungal agent. We often use antibacterial products thinking that we are protecting ourselves and our families from harmful germs. When we see a product that kills "99.95 percent of germs," it sounds like it's a good thing! Is it too good to be true? Most likely. Most of these products contain triclosan, which is found in everything from deodorant to antibacterial soaps and handwash, dishwashing liquid, socks and clothing, cutting boards, and even toothpaste. But did you know that triclosan is a pesticide? A 2017 study by the American Chemical Society also found that triclosan accumulates on the bristles of the toothbrush, prolonging exposure.[23]

Triclosan acts as an endocrine disruptor in the body. Exposure to triclosan can begin at birth; it has been found in three out of five samples of human breast milk.[24] Another problem is that it can contribute to antibiotic-resistant "superbugs."[25] Triclosan was originally used as a surgical scrub and in hospitals to prevent infections, but there is no data to show effectiveness when used in products found in a normal household.[26]

There is also evidence that suggests use of antibacterial products kills off normal bacteria while leaving tougher bacteria behind. The concern with that is the possibility of creating resistant bacteria. Triclosan has also been found to react with chlorine in tap water to form chloroform, a probable human carcinogen. Researchers at Virginia Polytechnic Institute studied triclosan using products such as soap and dishwashing products and found that the combination produced chloroform levels that met or exceeded the EPA's allowable amount.[27] The CDC states in its occupational health guidelines for chloroform that exposure to chloroform vapors can result in kidney and liver damage.

Antibacterial products do have their place, especially in hospitals, but their widespread use may be contributing to health problems as well as more illnesses that are resistant to the antibiotics used to treat them. Triclosan has even been banned in Minnesota, and the FDA states on its website that soaps containing antibacterial compounds like triclosan have not been shown to be "any more effective at preventing illness than washing with plain soap and water."[28] Many toothpaste brands have removed triclosan from their products, but in some instances, you will still find it. For all the reasons I've explained, I recommend you avoid triclosan in toothpaste as well as in other products, which we will review later in this section. Toothpaste can also contain other harmful ingredients like artificial sweeteners, carrageenan, SLS, and diethanolamine (DEA). When you shop for toothpaste, check the list of ingredients, and avoid all these substances. For a complete list of safer toothpaste brands, check the list of safer brands in the Resources section.

TOXIC CHEMICALS LURKING IN YOUR TOOTHPASTE

→ Triclosan (an endocrine disruptor)

→ SLS (an insecticide that can be contaminated with 1,4-dioxane, a carcinogenic byproduct

→ Artificial sweeteners

→ Carrageenan

→ DEA (another endocrine disruptor; also linked to cancer)

TEN MINUTES TO TOXIN-FREE TEETH

Go through your bathroom and examine your toothpaste labels.

→ Check for any of the ingredients listed in the previous list, "Toxic Chemicals Lurking in Your Toothpaste."

→ Replace your toothpaste with one from the list of safer brands in the Resources section.

→ DONE! See? It's easy and fun, and you'll feel so much better when your kids brush their teeth, you might even forget how many times you had to nag them to do it!

Fragrance

It makes a lot of sense that cosmetics are filled with nice scents—who doesn't like to smell fresh? Consumer research shows that scent is a key factor in a consumer's purchase decision-making process.[29] If a product smells like a gym locker, you can be sure it won't fly off the shelves. And if you've ever tried to use a nontoxic deodorant or sunscreen only to find that you smell like a pile of dirty laundry, now you know why: fragrance. (Or, in this case, lack thereof!)

Have you ever wondered what fragrance really is? Fragrance is considered to be a proprietary blend or a trade secret, so it's not required to be listed on labels. And it can be made up of anywhere from ten to over one hundred different chemicals, depending on the formulation. The annual sales of the fragrance and flavor industry was estimated at $22 billion in 2018 and expected to grow to $31 billion by 2026.[30] The industry is largely made up of four major companies.[31] The way your perfume is created to smell fresh is not all that different from how the butter on your popcorn is designed.[32] The International Fragrance Association lists approximately three thousand different stock chemicals that are used by its members to make up a fragrance formulation.[33] These chemicals include benzene derivatives as well as formaldehyde and other chemicals. These chemicals also include those that act as allergens, respiratory irritants, carcinogens, endocrine disruptors, and neurotoxic chemicals. Essentially, when you see the ingredient "fragrance," it can include a variety of chemicals that cause all sorts of serious health problems.

Fragrance was named "allergen of the year" in 2007 by the American Contact Dermatitis Society, and it's still considered to be one of the top five allergens.[34] You will also see it listed as "parfum," which sounds fancy, French, and *naturale*. Parfum often shows up in baby products that *look* natural and mild. But as far as I'm concerned, that "parfum" label could just say "made with up to one hundred unknown chemicals that haven't been tested for human safety." Doesn't sound quite so Parisian and carefree now, does it? The challenge with parfum, like so many of these toxins, is that it's very prevalent in cosmetics.

In case you live by Coco Chanel's famous words, "A woman who doesn't wear perfume has no future," I even have a slightly greener tip for you. I wouldn't deny anyone of a perfume spritz before date night or a special occasion—feel free to indulge every once in a while. For everyday wear, though, you can create your own blend from essential oils. Or if DIY is not your thing, you can buy perfume from companies that have natural blends such as Aftelier Perfumes or Kate's Magik. I also recommend checking out the Natural Perfumers Guild, a great

resource with links to brands that are certified natural perfumers selling naturally scented cologne.

THREE TIPS FOR SAFE PERFUME

1.   DIY! Perfume is easy to make from essential oils.

2.   Buy a safer brand from the Natural Perfumers Guild.

3.   If you can't part with your favorite perfume, save it for special occa-
      sions and not daily use.

Fragrance is in almost everything, so I don't want you to go to
the store and think, "It's too hard. I can't avoid it, so I'm not going to
try." If you can reduce exposure as much as possible, that's a *huge* step
forward. These incremental changes will make a difference in your
overall toxic load. Start by paying attention, slowly replacing products with parfum or fragrance, or using them sparingly.

SLIGHTLY LESS FRAGRANCE

→ Think of the top two personal care products that you use most often
   (lotion, shampoo, etc.).

→ Check the labels, and look for fragrance.

→ If the product has fragrance, replace it with a safer brand from the
   Resources section.

→ Optional: Save the fragrance-filled product for use on special occasions.

Here's another *slightly* greener tip that you can implement right
now: take your top two or three products with fragrance—the ones

you use most commonly or consume most often, like daily lotion or shampoo—and replace them with a product from the safer brands list in the Resources section.

Hidden toxins

There's another fun challenge with personal care products: some of the worst toxins aren't listed on product labels at all. These are what I call "hidden toxins"—ingredients that often contaminate a product but aren't required to be listed on the label because they haven't technically been added directly. Instead, they are byproducts of the manufacturing process or chemicals that appear in the cosmetic over time as the formula breaks down. There are two main categories of hidden toxins that we can look for and avoid in cosmetics: 1,4-dioxane and formaldehyde releasers. Though you won't see those exact terms on the label (since they are hidden!), I will teach you which ingredients to look for on the label that indicate their presence.

1,4-dioxane

This chemical is considered to be a byproduct of the manufacturing process, so it's not required to be listed on ingredient labels. It is created through a process called *ethoxylation*, where ethylene oxide is added to other chemicals to make them less harsh. For example, sodium lauryl sulfate, which is in many of our personal care products, such as shampoo and toothpaste, is known to be harsh and irritating to the skin. To make it less harsh, it is converted into sodium *laureth* sulfate through a process called ethoxylation.

The process, using ethylene oxide, and the reaction with the other chemicals produces small amounts of 1,4-dioxane. And because it is a byproduct of the manufacturing process and was not added to the product directly, 1,4-dioxane doesn't have to be listed on ingredient labels. It is listed by the California EPA as a suspected neurotoxicant (meaning that it's toxic to the nervous system) and has also been found to be toxic to the liver, kidneys, and respiratory system.[35] It is also listed by several sources, such as the EPA, the International Agency for Research on Cancer, and the Department of Health and Human Services as a probable human carcinogen. Ingredients that can create 1,4-dioxane include sodium laureth sulfate; polyethylene glycol (usually seen as PEG on labels); polysorbate 20, 60, and 80; phenoxyethanol; and ingredients that contain the words *oxynol*, *myreth*, *ceteareth*, *laureth*, *steareth*, and *oleth*.

When scanning labels for ingredients that may be contaminated with 1,4-dioxane, a quick tip for remembering ingredients is to look for things that end in *-eth*. So look for anything that says sodium laureth, PEG, or any polysorbate ingredient (followed by a number, such as 20, 60, or 80).

Formaldehyde releasers

Formaldehyde is a known cancer causer in humans, and it's also linked to organ and respiratory damage. Formaldehyde releasers are chemicals used in cosmetics that decompose slowly over time to produce and release formaldehyde, which acts a preservative for personal care products and cosmetics so that the product lasts longer. It's a simple technicality: once formaldehyde is released into the product, it now exists in the product, and you will be exposed. To avoid formaldehyde releasers in your cosmetics, don't buy products that contain DMDM hydantoin, quaternium-15, diazolidinyl urea, or imidazolidinyl urea. Look for these ingredients in personal care and beauty products such as shampoo and conditioners, lotions, shaving creams, sunscreen, baby shampoo, toothpaste, and liquid soap.

Slightly greener cosmetic shopping

As you shop for new cosmetics or when you are buying new lotions, creams, or sunscreen, remember just two things as you scan the label.

First, if you see an ingredient that ends in *-eth*, don't buy it.

Second, if you see any formaldehyde releasers (which include DMDM hydantoin, quaternium-15, diazolidinyl urea, and imidazolidinyl urea), stay away!

1,4-DIOXANE

What It Is

A trace contaminant that forms as a byproduct during the manufacturing process of certain cosmetic ingredients and is toxic to the liver, kidneys, and respiratory system.

Where It's Found

In cosmetics and personal care products, such as baby wash, bubble bath, shaving cream, shampoo, toothpaste, soaps, and more.

How to Avoid It

Look for these terms on the label:

→ Sodium laureth sulfate

→ Polyethylene glycol (PEG)

→ Polysorbate 20

→ Polysorbate 60

→ Polysorbate 80

→ Any other ingredients containing the words *oxynol*, *myreth*, *ceteareth*, *laureth*, *steareth*, and *oleth*

FORMALDEHYDE RELEASERS

What They Are

Chemicals used in cosmetics that decompose slowly over time to produce formaldehyde, which acts as a preservative.

Where They're Found

In nail polish, baby wash, bubble bath, shampoo/hair care products, shaving cream, body wash, baby wipes, and sunscreen.

How to Avoid Them

Look for these terms on the label:

→ DMDM hydantoin

→ Quaternium-15

→ Imidazolidinyl urea

→ Diazolidinyl urea

→ Sodium hydroxymethylglycinate

→ 2-bromo-2-nitropropane-1,3-diol (may be listed as "bronopol" on the label)

Buy nail polish that is labeled as "formaldehyde-free."

Toss/replace expired cosmetics.

Store cosmetics away from heat and light.

Another quick and easy tip I give people when they begin over-hauling their cosmetics is to replace their lip balm. Like toothpaste, lip balm can give us more exposure to harmful ingredients because it lands on (and in) our mouths. Even though we don't purposely ingest it, it's likely that some of it ends up in our mouths when we lick our lips, drink beverages, or eat food.

Traditional lip balm (the kind you see in tubes at the gro-cery, the pharmacy, or the gas station) contains all kinds of harm-ful chemicals. This is upsetting when you consider it's a product designed to go directly on your (or your kids') lips! The worst ingre-dients you will commonly see include paraffin, phenoxyethanol, flavor, and parabens. We will dig into parabens a bit later in this section, and you already know that flavor can contain hidden chem-icals. So let's review the health problems associated with paraffin and phenoxyethanol.

Paraffin can include contamination from ethylene oxide (a known cancer causer) and possibly 1,4-dioxane—a probable human carcino-gen, as we've discussed. So that's a *hard pass* from me. Phenoxyethanol is considered by the European Union to be toxic in products used in the mouth area.[36] The FDA stated in a press release that it "can depress the central nervous system and may cause vomiting and diarrhea."[37] (That might be worse than chapped lips.) It's also been known to cause allergic reactions, and several animal studies have shown it is toxic to the brain and nervous system.[38]

Another type of lip balm to be on the lookout for is medicated lip balm. In addition to the harmful ingredients we've already discussed, some medicated lip balms also contain phenol. Phenol exposure can occur from medicated products such as ear drops, throat drops, and mouthwash as well as through medicated lip balms. The EPA states that phenol is considered to be quite toxic to humans via oral exposure.[39] Not that we usually run around eating tubes of lip balm, but it is certainly easy to ingest it through licking lips or while drinking and eating soon after applying. It's especially tough for kids not to lick their lips when they are wearing delicious-smelling cherry lip balm!

Phenol has also been listed as a neurotoxin (again, that's a chemical known to cause toxicity to the brain) and to have "adverse effects on the human nervous system" by environmental medicine doctors Philippe Grandjean and Philip Landrigan.[40] It has also been found to cause adverse nervous system effects such as lethargy, seizures, muscle weakness, and vertigo.[41]

Even though I tend to use my kitchen more frequently for conversation than for cooking, I *do* like to whip up a batch of homemade lip balm every now and then. While the initial investment may seem more expensive, you can make a huge number of lip balms—and other simple DIY recipes—from a few simple ingredients. Homemade lip balm is a fraction of the cost of the store-bought kind. Plus, you can keep remaking these anytime you need them, or better yet, try out more DIY recipes! Many DIY skin care recipes use the same ingredients, so if you like the DIY lifestyle, your leftover supply won't go to waste. If you still think making your cosmetics sounds pretty daunting, I promise it's easier than making a grilled cheese sandwich.

DIY RECIPE FOR LIP BALM

Here's what you'll need.

Equipment

Double boiler*

Pipettes for pouring (two options: glass or plastic. I prefer glass.)

Chap stick tubes

*   *Can also add water to a larger pot and place a slightly smaller pot on top to add ingredients to if you don't have a double boiler.*

Ingredients

4 tablespoons organic coconut oil

2 tablespoons shea butter

6 teaspoons beeswax

2–3 drops vitamin E oil

Directions

Melt the coconut oil, shea butter, and beeswax over low heat in the double boiler, stirring frequently. Remove from heat and add 1–2 drops vitamin E oil—don't add too much unless you want a lip gloss look! Whisk together quickly before it hardens. Use the pipettes to pour the mixture into tubes. Put them into the fridge to cool and harden when finished.

Makes approximately 12–14 tubes.

INGREDIENTS TO AVOID IN LIP BALM

→ Paraffin

→ Phenoxyethanol

→ Phenol

→ Flavor

→ Parabens

Other ingredients to avoid

Now we will dig into some of the other ingredients I recommend you avoid in personal care products, including ethanolamines, mineral oil, and SLS. These chemicals are added to lengthen the shelf life of the product, create foam, thicken the formula, or keep the ingredients mixed together. Even mild baby products can contain ingredients that are problematic. I always figured that products formulated for a baby would be absolutely safe, but that's not always so! Now I know better and look more closely at what the product is made with.

DEA, MEA, TEA

Let's talk about ethanolamines. (Try saying that ten times fast!) You'll typically find these listed as DEA, MEA, or TEA on product labels. These are chemically modified forms of coconut oil that act as thickening and foaming agents, and they're used in many personal care and beauty products. They're also used to help oil-soluble and water-soluble ingredients blend together. They're typically found in things that foam, such as soaps, shampoos, shaving creams, liquid hand soaps, and baby wash as well as cosmetics such as mascara, eye shadow, blush, foundation, conditioners, fragrance, and sunscreens.

DEA, MEA, and TEA are linked to liver tumors and can be contaminated with nitrosamines, which are impurities that can show up in a wide variety of ingredients and are known to cause cancer.[42] Because they're considered impurities, nitrosamines are not required to be listed on product labels.

Mineral oil

When you first look at the name "mineral oil," it seems pretty harmless. It sounds like an oil that comes from minerals. What's wrong with that? Mineral oil is a colorless, odorless oil that's made from petroleum as a byproduct of the distillation to produce gasoline. It's used in creams, lotions, eye shadow, lip gloss, hair products, lipstick, blush, concealer, and baby oil. While the technical grade mineral oil that is used as an engine lubricant is a known human cancer causer, the type of mineral oil that's used in cosmetics is more purified.

But this type of mineral oil is still derived from petroleum, which means there can be contamination with cancer-causing hydrocarbons during the refining process. Hydrocarbons are chemical mixtures that come from crude oil.[43] A study in the *Journal of Women's Health* stated that there is strong evidence that mineral oil hydrocarbons are the greatest contaminant in the human body.[44] Why are mineral oil hydrocarbons so prevalent? They are widely found not only in cosmetics but also in the air we breathe as well as in food packaging.[45]

In that *Journal of Women's Health* study, researchers sought to identify the most relevant sources of mineral oil contamination. To do that, they removed fat specimens from women who had cesarean sections and collected milk samples from women after they gave birth. The scientists found that both the fat and the milk samples were contaminated with mineral oil. In fact, they were saturated with hydrocarbons. They also determined that the increase in mineral oil contamination in the human fat tissue suggests an accumulation over time and that cosmetics might be a relevant source of the contamination. So *mineral oil* is a bit of a misnomer, because to me, it sounds pretty harmless.

The molecular mass of mineral oil reabsorbed by our body is higher than assumed by the safety evaluation of the European Food Safety Authority, and that causes health risks.[46] Scientists are concerned that much of the mineral oil we are exposed to on a daily basis does contain contaminants that could affect our health and that it has not been convincingly shown that these contaminants can be tolerated without health concerns in humans. An editorial in the *European Journal of Lipid Science and Technology* concluded that the safety of human exposure to mineral oil needs to be proven, or we have to take measures to reduce our exposure from all sources, including cosmetics.[47] Another health concern associated with mineral oil is that it is comedogenic, which means that it clogs pores, forming a physical barrier to reduce moisture loss in skin. This barrier can inhibit the skin's own oil production and also prevent the release of toxins through the skin.

Sodium lauryl sulfate

When we talked about toothpaste earlier, I mentioned the chemical sodium lauryl sulfate or SLS. You may also see sodium laureth sulfate, also known as SLES, on product labels. They're both found in many personal care and beauty products as well as cleaning products. Soaps, shampoos, bubble bath, toothpaste, body wash, baby wash, shaving cream, mouthwash, and face cleaners commonly contain SLS. It is added to cosmetics and cleaning products as an emulsifier to help keep ingredients mixed and also as a surfactant to get rid of dirt and grime and help clean as well as to make things foam. A surfactant is a component of most cleaning detergents—it stirs up dirt on the surface so it can be trapped and lifted up.

SLS can be manufactured in a laboratory setting, or it can originate from natural sources like coconuts or palm kernel oil.[48] But the process it goes through to create foam makes it anything but natural. SLES is the result of SLS undergoing a process called *ethoxylation*, which is done to make SLS less harsh and irritating. This process uses ethylene oxide, which is a known human carcinogen.[49] It has been shown to harm the nervous system, and it is categorized by the California EPA as a possible developmental toxicant based on evidence that it may interfere with human development. *Super scary.* SLS also does damage by stripping skin of its protective oils and moisture. In fact, SLS is a model substance in testing skin irritability in lab testing. This means researchers who are testing skin healing products use SLS as an intentionally irritating agent. First they irritate the skin with SLS, and then they test the effectiveness of their new products intended to heal the skin.[50]

SLS is also linked to hair loss when used in shampoos and other hair care products, because it can be so irritating to skin and hair follicles. It has even been shown to slow hair growth, and it is also a detergent and therefore quite drying to hair and potentially leading to breakage.

A study in Norway found that toothpaste containing SLS is associated with an increase in canker sores in the mouth, likely due to weakening and irritation of the oral mucosa. This weakening exposes the oral epithelium—a lower low layer of skin—making it more exposed and vulnerable to irritants.[51] The results of this study found a significant reduction in canker sores when study participants brushed with an SLS-free toothpaste.

A second problem with SLES is that the ethoxylation process can also produce 1,4-dioxane as a byproduct. If you recall from earlier in this chapter, 1,4-dioxane is a probable human carcinogen.[52] It's also one of those sneaky toxins I mentioned. Now, it is *possible* that 1,4-dioxane can be removed from cosmetics during the manufacturing process by vacuum stripping it. This is a process where the solution is heated using steam, and a vacuum is used to suck out a particular ingredient. But there is no easy way to know whether products containing SLES have actually undergone this process. And even if the product has been vacuum stripped, a residue can remain.[53] So in my opinion, it's safer to avoid this ingredient as much as possible.

There are also a couple more related ingredients that I've seen on labels lately too: ammonium lauryl sulfate and ammonium laureth sulfate. Both of these have similar health concerns to SLS and SLES, and I recommend avoiding them as well.

FIVE ALL-NATURAL HAIR TIPS AND TRICKS

1. Rinse with apple cider vinegar for shiny hair. Pour half a cup of apple cider vinegar onto hair and scalp after shampooing and conditioning and then rinse. Don't worry. The smell fades quickly!

2. Condition hair with avocado, olive oil, and coconut oil. Mix about a quarter of a cup of olive oil and two tablespoons of coconut oil in a bowl, then mash in several slices of avocado (you can adjust these measurements according to the length of your hair). Once the avocado is mashed in, pull your hair into a ponytail and spread the mixture the length of the ponytail, concentrating on the ends. Wrap your hair in a towel and leave on for at least thirty minutes. Use once a week. *Tips:* Put a small amount of conditioner on your ponytail first to help wash the oils out. You may want to put a plastic shower cap on first to protect the towel.

3. Add essential oils linked to hair growth to your shampoo. These include lavender, cedarwood, peppermint, cypress, clary sage, Roman chamomile, and rosemary. Add just a couple of drops, and shake the bottle well before each use.

4. Healthy hair growth mask #1: Pour jojoba oil into a two-ounce glass dropper bottle, and add approximately six to eight drops each of cedarwood, Roman chamomile, clary sage, and rosemary essential oils. Massage well into scalp, then wrap with a towel and leave on for a couple of hours. You can also cover your pillow with a towel and sleep with the mask on overnight. *Tip*: This goes on better with slightly damp hair. Use one to two times per week.

5. Healthy hair growth mask #2: Mix two tablespoons of apple cider

vinegar, half a ripe avocado, and one egg yolk in a bowl. Blend until
smooth and the consistency of a paste. Rub the mask into your hair,
then place a shower cap on your head, followed by a towel, and
leave on for a couple of hours. Use one to two times per week.

Methylisothiazolinone

Methylisothiazolinone, also known as MIT, is a preservative used
in personal care and cleaning products. It is found in things such
as shampoos, baby wipes, sunscreens, and moisturizers. Tests have
shown it to be a neurotoxin.[54] It can also be toxic to the immune
system, potentially leading to allergies and asthma, autoimmune conditions, and cancer.[55] The EWG lists MIT as an allergen and as being
toxic to human skin.[56] In fact, it was named "allergen of the year" in
2013 by the American Contact Dermatitis Society, which is a designation used to draw attention to the agents causing the most significant
negative clinical effects.[57] MIT is being used more and more exten-
sively in products, even though there have been no neurotoxicity studies performed to see what exposure level is safe for humans. Dr. Elias
Aizenman, professor of neurobiology at the University of Pittsburgh
School of Medicine, became concerned about MIT when he realized
that despite its widespread use in consumer products, there was no
research about its potential neurotoxic effects on humans. He was
particularly concerned about the possible impact on developing
fetuses. Dr. Aizenman says that while additional research needs to
be done, he believes it's possible there could be a connection between
higher exposures to MIT and the noticeably higher rates of diagnosed

developmental disabilities, such as ADHD, learning disabilities, and autism.[58]

A European safety committee has said that MIT should be used only in limited quantities for rinse-off products like soaps and shampoos and that no safe concentrations exists for leave-on products like lotions, even though it is found in these types of products.[59] Some studies have also shown that the levels allowed in rinse-off products may still be too high. To identify it, I always skim the label until I see the "methyl." And if I locate that, I then look for the "thiaz." Another tip I've discovered is that it's usually found toward the end of the ingredient list.

The bottom line

Until the FDA drastically changes the way it regulates cosmetics, it's on us as consumers to educate and inform ourselves about what we are putting on our kids' skin as well as on our own. It's important to limit our exposure to these dangerous chemicals at least *some* of the time, especially for kids who are at increased risk. I suggest you start with toothpaste, making sure that the brand you use is safe, and add on and build from there. Next, make sure your lip balm is safe, and avoid products that contain fragrance. Finally, look for hidden toxins lurking in your cosmetics (formaldehyde releasers and 1,4-dioxane), and carry the list of toxins to avoid in cosmetics with you when you go shopping. Most of my clients find that once they've done this one or two times, they know exactly which ingredients to avoid going forward, and the process becomes second nature.

8

Change Your Body Wash and Lose Weight

"I saw your article about toothpaste containing stuff that might keep us fat," a woman named Miranda wrote to me on Facebook, "so I decided to avoid antibacterial products, parabens, and fragrance in my beauty routine. All my friends thought I was crazy for throwing out most of my products. I live in New York City and am on a pretty tight budget. But even with the snow and the cold this winter, I looked and felt amazing! Thank you so much for posting your advice online. Just by removing those ingredients, I was able to reduce my body fat percentage by 3 percent! And I didn't get sick from riding the subway like I used to either. I'm happily slightly greener...and *definitely* more than slightly skinnier!"

Miranda's story is not uncommon. As we discovered in the previous chapter, most personal care products—including soaps, body washes, shampoos, conditioners, hair products, cosmetics, and even toothpaste, mouthwash, and floss—contain chemicals that disrupt our body's natural hormones. Some parabens and phthalates and triclosan have been labeled *obesogens*, which are a particular type of endocrine disruptor that can cause weight gain. Not all endocrine disruptors are obesogens, but all obesogens *are* disruptive and can make us gain weight.

But wait, this is the cosmetics section, not the food section. Is this really where a conversation about weight gain belongs? Yep! While there are some obesogens in food and other ingredients like MSG that can cause us to gain weight (either by suppressing that full feeling or by disrupting our hormones), we tend to get more exposure to them through our personal care products. And the negative impact that obesogens have on our weight gain, while unfortunate, is not nearly as profound as the impact it has on our kids, especially prenatally. Some researchers even believe that obesogen exposure in utero can have a multigenerational effect, putting your *grandchildren* at risk of greater susceptibility to obesity. Some scientists wonder if the stark rise we're seeing in obesity today might be connected to chemical exposure a couple of generations back. We can't do anything about what our grandmothers did or didn't do, ate or didn't eat, but since emerging research shows that there could be a connection, it pays to limit our toxin exposure. There's research to back up this moderate (a.k.a. slightly greener) approach.

COMMON ENDOCRINE DISRUPTORS IN COSMETICS

→ Phthalates

→ Fragrance

→ Triclosan

→ Parabens

Where They're Found

→ Personal care products such as hair products, body wash, lotion, deodorant, shave creams, antiaging moisturizers, toothpaste, and antibacterial soaps and hand sanitizer

→ Cosmetics, such as eye shadow, lipstick, foundation, and lip balm

What are obesogens?

Endocrine disruptors were first discovered in 1991, when scientists realized that environmental toxins could negatively affect the endocrine system. About a decade later, a researcher named Dr. Paula Baillie-Hamilton found that environmental chemicals could play a role in fat cell development and might be connected to obesity.[1] In 2006, a researcher named Dr. Bruce Blumberg officially coined the term *obesogen* for a chemical that could cause weight gain and lead to obesity. Before that time, it was believed that weight maintenance followed a pretty simple formula: weight gain (or loss) = calories consumed—calories burned. Maintaining body weight, while often difficult, was viewed through a simple lens: if you eat too much and don't exercise enough, you'll gain weight.

If you think about it, it makes sense that chemicals can play a role in how the body maintains weight. Have you ever taken a medication that came with a side effect of gaining weight? Birth control pills, antidepressants, other psychiatric medications...

there have long been medications that come with weight gain as a known side effect. Scientists used to believe that fat cells stored or released energy based on how much energy the body consumed or expended, but now, they have learned that the functionality of human fat cells isn't quite that simple! Fat cells are actually complex glands that can communicate with other tissues, like the brain and the immune system. Of course, your weight isn't static, and you're never stuck with it; you can always exercise or eat healthier, and your fat cells will likely become smaller. But if your body has been "programmed" to develop more fat cells, it *can* make staying at a healthy weight even harder. Today, there are about fifty known (or potential) obesogens, but researchers are only just beginning to understand the full scope of how they affect us. What we do know is that there *are* some pretty simple ways to reduce your exposure and that doing so is important and impactful. In this chapter, you will learn exactly which ingredients to avoid in your personal care products, where you'll find them, and—as always—which safer brands you can replace them with.

But first, let's take an even closer look at what happens when we are exposed to obesogens.

How obesogens affect us before birth

Studies have found that both obesity and metabolic syndrome can be preprogrammed in utero during development through the mother's exposure to toxins.[2] Metabolic syndrome is a set of conditions (high blood pressure, high blood sugar, excess body fat around the waist, and abnormal cholesterol or triglyceride levels) that increase the risk of heart disease, stroke, and type 2 diabetes.[3]

While it was long thought that obesity—or even just struggling to maintain your weight—was primarily a problem of adulthood, emerging research is proving that slowing metabolism in older age may not be the only factor. Of course, this doesn't justify frequent triple scoop ice creams or coffees piled with whipped cream or offer a hall pass to sit on the couch all day, but it does mean that there are environmental factors that explain the rise in obesity. For some people, the struggle to maintain weight can be traced back to their time in their mother's womb. Some researchers believe that obesogens are the reason for the rise in obesity for children and in people under the age of fifty, when these chemicals became more common and exposure during development was more likely. Scientists are also delving into more research around what's called "transgenerational inheritance," meaning they are seeking to understand to what extent obesogen exposure can impact future generations.

How do obesogens cause us to gain weight?

There are several different ways that obesogens affect weight. Some of them can cause us to have more fat cells, larger fat cells, fat cells that store more fat, or all three, none of which we want, of course![4] Other obesogens can interfere with the hormones that regulate our metabolism, changing the way our bodies create fatty tissue, altering our appetites and how full we feel, and even changing our food preferences. Obesogens can also affect energy balance, causing our bodies to store more calories, and affect organs like the pancreas, liver, gastrointestinal tract, muscles, and brain. Obesogens can potentially cause unwanted changes in these tissues and how they instruct insulin sensitivity and fat metabolism.

As you can see, the changes obesogens can make to our delicate hormonal systems are complex and can literally affect almost the whole body as it relates to weight maintenance. The effects that obesogens have can vary from person to person—something that's true of most environmental toxins. We probably all have that one friend who says, "Well, my uncle Peter smoked three packs a day, guzzled whiskey, and still lived to be ninety-five years old." Every data set has outliers! And if you recall sixth-grade math, outliers are the exception and not the rule. Toxins tend to impact people differently. But until there's a blood test that can say, "Tonya, you're the one person who is not affected by obesogens!" data suggests that reducing our exposure is the wisest choice.

HOW DO OBESOGENS CAUSE WEIGHT GAIN?

→ They disrupt metabolism.

→ They increase the size and number of fat cells.

→ They affect thyroid function.

→ They alter appetite and satiety (feeling full or satisfied after eating).

→ They accumulate in the body (in fat cells).

What can we do?

While it's next to impossible to avoid obesogens completely, the good news is there are definitely things we can do to reduce our exposure. If you can choose one or two of the most frequently used personal care products in your home that contain obesogens and replace those with a safer brand, you're already making a positive impact. Choosing products that don't contain these chemicals as often as possible can greatly reduce your exposure (and maybe your waistline) while also improving the health of your family and possibly that of future generations too.

Now we will go through some of the obesogens frequently found in cosmetic products, and I will explain exactly what to look for and how to avoid them. Then, we will review the rest of the ingredients I recommend avoiding in personal care products. We will also talk about sunscreen, which tends to have some other harmful ingredients that I recommend you avoid when possible.

Obesogen #1: Parabens

Parabens are used as preservatives to prevent the growth of bacteria and have been popular since the 1920s to extend the shelf life of beauty products. They are found in tons of products—everything from deodorants and shampoos to conditioners, sunscreens, hairstyling gels, and shaving gels and lotions. Most commonly, you will see butylparaben, ethylparaben, propylparaben, and methylparaben. Every once in a while they're labeled as *isobutylparaben* or *isopropylparaben*. Sometimes a single product contains multiple parabens.

A study consisting of several groups of researchers, including ones from the Centers for Disease Control, and published in the September 2014 *Journal of Epidemiology* found that exposure to certain substances, such as triclosan and parabens, may disrupt boys' growth during their fetal development and the first years of life.[5] This particular study was specifically designed to study the health effects in one gender—in this case, male—because of the differences between the two sexes. Paraben exposure was also associated with an increased weight at birth and at three years old. It's also known that accelerated growth in the first years of life can lead to an increased risk of obesity later in childhood.[6] Researchers have said they will try to repeat these results in a future study to see if they can find when these substances have the greatest influence on development, and they also plan on including girls in the study as well, since their sensitivity to parabens may be different.

Parabens are also linked to breast cancer. You may have heard of this study in the *Journal of Applied Toxicology*—as it received media attention—that revealed that up to six different types of parabens have been found in the tissue of biopsied breast cancer tumors.[7] Many studies have confirmed that estrogen plays a central role in the development, progression, and treatment of breast cancer, and parabens have been shown to mimic estrogen.[8] What that means is that parabens can penetrate the skin and act like a weak form of estrogen in the body, potentially switching on the development of hormone-receptor-positive breast cancers.[9] This also brings up the question of what happens when environmental chemicals such as parabens enter the breast and mimic estrogen action. In fact, another study found parabens can actually promote the growth of estrogen-sensitive breast tumors, even in tiny amounts.[10]

One piece of good news: parabens are cleared from the body pretty quickly.[11] But the bad news is we're exposed to parabens through so many products that we almost always have them in our systems. However, there are many great alternatives now that are paraben-free, so it's easy to change how you shop and improve your health! Many companies are getting the message to remove toxic chemicals and are changing formulations due to consumer demand.

Obesogen #2: Triclosan

Triclosan is an antibacterial ingredient that is commonly found in toothpaste. I'd like to dig into some of the science here behind why I recommend you avoid it in other products, including hand sanitizer, deodorants, high chair trays, school supplies such as pencils, clothing, hand soaps, cosmetics, mouthwash, dish soap, cutting boards, and toothbrushes. One animal study showed a potential increase in skin cancer risk after long-term exposure to triclosan.[12] Another study is underway to determine if triclosan might break down into other chemicals in human skin when exposed to UV rays from the sun. The FDA ruled that hand soap and body washes that contain triclosan aren't allowed to be introduced or marketed after September 6, 2017, along with nineteen other antibacterial ingredients, including triclocarban, which is a close chemical relative of triclosan. This ruling applies to over-the-counter hand soaps and body washes for household use, but it doesn't apply to hand sanitizers. So if you want to avoid triclosan, look for it on hand sanitizer ingredient labels. And remember, the FDA has stated that washing your hands with regular soap and water is just as effective!

HOW TO AVOID TRICLOSAN

Avoid products with triclosan on the label, and watch for these other names for it:

→ Irgasan

→ Lexol 300

→ Ster-Zac

→ Triclocarban

→ Additive B

→ Cloxifenolum

Avoid these brand names:

→ Microban

→ BioFresh

Obesogen #3: Phthalates

Phthalates are chemicals often added to plastics to make them more flexible, but you'll also find them in many personal care products where they perform different functions such as keeping mascara from running and helping fragrances last longer. They're normally unlabeled, sometimes hiding under the term *other* or *fragrance*. If they are listed, you'll see them as DBT, DEP, or DEHP. Phthalates are a probable human carcinogen.[13] They act as endocrine disruptors. They have also been linked to reduced IQ in children who have had prenatal exposure.[14]

A study on phthalate exposure in children found that phthalate levels in the kids tested were higher those than of adults in a similar study.[15] We'll address this in more depth later on—when we talk about reducing toxins beyond the kitchen and the bathroom—but one possible reason for this is because children are so closely tied to their environment. Children play on the floor and lick their fingers, and because phthalates can be found in everything from personal care products to vinyl shower curtains and laminate flooring, it's easier for them to pick up exposure. A lot of soaps contain phthalates too, so I use castile soap for everything. I especially love Dr. Bronner's and Vermont Soap Organics. If you have trouble finding these products in your local supermarket, try shopping online at Vitacost or Thrive Market, both of which I highly recommend. They have great prices and great selections, but not everything they carry is organic and free of toxic chemicals, so you have to check the labels carefully, just as you would in a regular grocery store.

Surprising facts about sunscreen

After we cover obesogens, I like to talk to clients about sunscreen and the hidden dangers within the sprays and lotions we put on our skin to "protect" us. When I first started researching the dangers of conventional sunscreen, I was shocked at how many toxic chemical ingredients are used in popular sunblock brands. I was most surprised to learn that some of those toxic chemicals could possibly become *even more toxic when they are exposed to sunlight.*

Wait, say that again? I know. Chemicals known to have worsening toxicity in the sun are used specifically in the sun. You can't make this stuff up! Not only are we harming ourselves by slathering it all over our skin, we are exposing our children to it. Their bodies are less able to handle toxins, and their skin readily absorbs them. If you do have to use sunscreen, buy one that is as natural as possible, and use it only when you have to be out for long periods of time during peak sun hours. While it is extremely important to protect our skin from excessive sun exposure to guard against skin cancer, studies have also shown that getting regular, smaller exposures to the sun without the use of sunscreen is important to our health, especially for the body's production of vitamin D.

Vitamin D and sun exposure

Your body's natural vitamin D production can be reduced by 97.5 to 99.9 percent when using sunscreen. Vitamin D deficiency is directly related to many different diseases, including heart disease, multiple sclerosis, rheumatoid arthritis, inflammatory bowel disease, cancer, and diabetes.[16] Vitamin D is made by the body with the help of sunlight, and this transformation takes place in the skin. Although vitamin D can be ingested through food, those levels may not be adequate for many people.

Vitamin D is also available in supplement form, but unless you know your actual vitamin D level, it is hard to gauge how much you really need. It is also important to remember that vitamins work synergistically rather than as isolated compounds, so getting direct sunlight is the most natural and beneficial way to maintain healthy vitamin D levels. Daily brief exposure to the sun is often enough for your body to produce adequate vitamin D.

According to the World Health Organization, five to fifteen minutes of sun exposure to the face, arms, and hands without sunscreen just two to three times a week can help with the synthesis of vitamin D to help keep levels sufficiently high.[17] Going outside early in the spring season and slowly increasing that time is a good approach for acclimating your skin to the sun without the use of sunscreen. If you do this, I also like to recommend avoiding the sun's peak sun hours of 10:00 a.m. to 4:00 p.m. to help you avoid the more dangerous sun exposure that causes sunburn.

During peak sun hours, consider staying in the shade or using protective clothing and a hat. Studies show that excess sun exposure that results in sunburn is a well-known risk factor for melanoma, a deadly form of skin cancer. Your risk of getting melanoma increases in relationship to sunburn frequency and severity. However, sun exposure without burning can decrease the chance of developing melanoma.[18]

One of the reasons for this has to do with ultraviolet (UV) rays. UV light comes in two main wavelengths: UVA and UVB. UVB is the light that helps your skin produce vitamin D, and UVA is the light that penetrates the skin more deeply, causing more damage from free radicals. UVA rays are constant throughout the entire day, while UVB rays are low in the morning and evening and high during midday.[19] The majority of sunscreens do not protect you from UVA rays, no matter how high the SPF, and instead filter out the somewhat more beneficial UVB rays that help produce vitamin D.

INGREDIENTS TO AVOID IN SUNSCREEN

These will be listed under "active ingredients" on sunscreen labels:

→ Avobenzone

→ Oxybenzone

→ Octinoxate

→ Octisalate

→ Homosalate

Harmful ingredients hiding in your sunscreen

When you do use sunscreen, choose an all-natural sunscreen to reduce your exposure to toxins. One of the main chemicals used in sunscreens to filter out UVB rays, octinoxate, was found to be especially toxic when exposed to sunlight, resulting in increased toxicity.[20] Researchers from one study suggested that octinoxate became twice as toxic in the sunlight as it was alone. It was also found to cause estrogenic effects in laboratory animals (estrogen disruptors are linked to breast and prostate cancer) as well as disruption of thyroid hormones and brain signaling.[21]

Oxybenzone is a one of the most common ingredients in commercial sunscreens. Studies have shown that it can cause skin allergies and can interfere with how some hormones work.[22] Two other ingredients, octinoxate and octisalate, are penetration enhancers, which may actually increase the amount of sunscreen ingredients that are absorbed into the skin, while another ingredient, homosalate, can enhance the penetration of the toxic herbicide 2,4-D (this is a component of Agent Orange and is commonly used to spray crops as well as turf and lawns).[23] This makes it an especially harmful sunscreen ingredient for those in the farming and ground maintenance industries and even for golfers who may use it on a golf course where 2,4-D may have been used.

These are some pretty scary facts, especially when it has been found that these chemicals are absorbed directly into the bloodstream. In general, I recommend using common sense: stay in the shade when possible, avoid getting sunburned, and choose a safer brand when it's necessary to wear sunscreen.

TOP FIVE TIPS FOR SUNSCREEN SAFETY

1.   Avoid sunscreens with harmful ingredients.

2.   Apply sunscreen fifteen minutes before heading outside. That's how long it can take to absorb into skin and do its work.

3.   Apply sunscreen liberally. Be sure to slather it on thickly.

4.   Reapply sunscreen throughout the day. Sunscreens are not meant for more than a couple of hours. Reapply frequently, especially after sweating or being in water, even with water-resistant sunscreen.

5.   Get in the shade whenever possible. If you'll be outside for hours at a time, sunscreen should not be your first line of defense.

After we've overhauled their personal care products, clients sometimes ask me what my skin care routine is, because it can start to feel like *everything* is off-limits. I like to remind people we don't necessarily need all these harsh chemicals to have healthy, vibrant skin. I ask them to consider the fact that a lot of our product purchases are driven by marketing. Personally, I wash with jojoba oil (sometimes with a cleanser to exfoliate), tone with a rose water spray, and follow with a serum. All these skin care products are made by one of my favorite brands, Green Envee.

TONYA'S SAFE SKIN CARE ROUTINE

→ Wash with jojoba oil.

→ Use a safe brand to exfoliate if you need to.

→ Tone with rose water spray.

→ Follow with a serum.

To review

There are lots of land mines out there when trying to determine which cosmetics are safe and what's really in them. Here's what I recommend:

1. Don't fall for false labels that are "dermatologist approved." Read the ingredients.
2. Avoid products with the most harmful ingredients:
   a. Formaldehyde releasers
   b. Parabens
   c. Fragrance/parfum
   d. Phthalates
   e. DEA, MEA, TEA
   f. 1,4-dioxane
   g. Triclosan

    h.   Sodium lauryl sulfate

    i.   Methylisothiazolinone

    j.   Mineral oil

3.   Start with toothpaste and lip balm, and replace those first!

4.   Use perfume or other "must have" cosmetics with harmful ingredients only on special occasions.

5.   Choose safer brands of sunscreen when it is necessary to use it.

In the next chapter, we will review cosmetic label reading in action, and we will complete the entire Slightly Greener Method cleanout. Hopefully by now, you've implemented one or two simple tricks that change the way you wear and use personal care products. Keep up the good work!

9

Reading Cosmetic Labels, Expiration Dates, and the Slightly Greener Cleanout

Now that you know which ingredients to avoid on cosmetic products, let's take a look at what label reading looks like in action. Shopping for shampoos, sunscreen, and makeup can be tricky. You'll often see "natural" sections in drugstores or cosmetic retail outlets. Even when you know to be skeptical of marketing claims, it can be tempting to get lured in by false promises. I've seen shampoo bottles with all white labels adorned with a sprig of lavender and felt tempted. My brain said, "Tonya, read the ingredients." But when I was just starting out developing the Slightly Greener Method, my impulses still tried to take over at times.

"I want that shampoo," my irrational mind said. It looked safe! But when I picked up the bottle, turned it around, and looked on the back...

Jiminy Cricket.

So many times, I wanted to throw that bottle on the ground, call up the founder of that company, and yell at them for trying to trick me. Because often on the back of that *oh-so-chic* label, I would see several of the very ingredients I've been teaching you to avoid. It's like the devil in sheep's clothing. Don't be fooled.

Label reading in action

To show just how deceiving cosmetic labels can be, my daughters Kaylee and Lyndsey and I took a trip to the local pharmacy to try reading product labels and implementing my label reading tips. We headed to a popular national retail chain and started out in the shampoo aisle. We were shocked to see how many of the "natural" and "fresh" shampoos were full of all the harmful chemicals I suggest you avoid.

Lyndsey picked up a shampoo bottle that said "repairs damaged hair" and "leaves hair restored." Who doesn't want that? But here's what we found on the back of that bottle, in the ingredients section:

- **Sodium laureth sulfate** ("-eth" means 1,4-dioxane contamination, which is a possible cancer causer)
- **Laureth-2** (another "-eth")
- **Laureth-4** (another "-eth")
- **Laureth-23** (another "-eth")
- **PEG-7** (another ingredient that could be contaminated with 1,4-dioxane, a probable cancer causer)
- **PEG 40** (another possible contamination with 1,4-dioxane)
- **PEG 120** (another possible contamination with 1,4-dioxane)

In just one shampoo bottle, we found *seven* different ingredients with possible contaminations. Then we picked up another shampoo; the label had roses and herbs on it and words like "smooth" and "fresh." Harmless, right?

Nope.

Right away on the back label, I spotted methylisothiazolinone—I always scan for that one. (Remember the trick: it's a long word that starts with an M, so I always look for that and the "methyl" first. Then I look for "thiazolinone"—it's an allergen and is also potentially linked to neurotoxicity and developmental issues.)

I always rule this one out, especially because we have ADHD and learning disabilities in our family. This product also had some yellow dye colors and fragrance. Another "moisturizing" shampoo had cocamidopropyl betaine, which can be contaminated with nitrosamines, known cancer causers. However, I finally did find a shampoo with safe ingredients, like honeysuckle flower extract, avocado oil, and aloe vera leaf juice—yay!

So the point is, you *can* find safe products, even at your local pharmacy or drug store. You just have to use my tricks for reading the labels carefully. Or, if you want to skip the whole label-reading process all together, you can just try a few of the safer brands I recommend and decide which one you like best! But once you use the label reading tricks a few times in practice, it really becomes second nature, and you don't have to worry so much about it.

Sadly, many if not most of the products we found didn't meet my safety standards. Kaylee picked up some lotion made by a popular brand, and the label said, "dermatologist recommended," "fragrance-free," and "soothing oatmeal." That sounded pretty good at first. But the ingredient label revealed something completely different. I found five different parabens listed in the ingredients: methylparaben, ethylparaben, butylparaben, propylparaben, and isobutylparaben.

Remember the problem with parabens? They've been found in the tissue of biopsied breast tumors, and they're very strong endocrine disruptors. They can also cause all sorts of problems and are linked to infertility in males, breast cancer, gestational diabetes in pregnant women, altered thyroid function, and the development of allergies and eczema.[1]

Next we picked up a popular sunscreen brand, and the particular bottle we chose was made specifically for babies. Of course, you would think, baby sunscreen is different from the adult version. Surely there is a safer version for the littlest humans? But the answer, sadly, is no. This particular sunscreen had two parabens in it as well as a formaldehyde releaser. So an unknowing parent would slather this sunscreen—which has two endocrine disruptors linked to breast cancer and a formaldehyde releaser that creates small doses of a known cancer causer—all over their tiny baby.

Hopefully the lesson here has become clear: whenever you shop for food, makeup, or other personal care products—anything that you're putting into or on your body—check the ingredient list. Savvy marketers and store owners will try every trick in the book to persuade you to make a purchase. Remember to focus on the ingredients, and you will be just fine.

A note on expiration dates

OK, now you're an ingredient sleuthing professional, and you know exactly what to look for on labels. You've selected a safer brand and brought your product home. Now you just use it until it runs out, right? Well, in some cases—like with most shampoos—yes. But in other cases—like mascara, eye shadow, and sunscreen—you need to toss it with the seasons.

Really? Makeup can expire? Yes, it can, and using expired makeup can, in some instances, cause health problems.

The problem with old makeup

When was the last time you found an old tube of concealer in a purse stored under your bed and thought: *Score!* It's almost like seeing a twenty-dollar bill on the ground. Finding a half-used lipstick can feel like discovering free cash.

But in many cases, you shouldn't use it.

A 2015 study found that most women know that makeup can go bad, but few follow the guidelines about when it should be thrown away.[2] That same survey asked over four thousand women about their purchasing habits and how they use makeup in their daily lives; 80 percent of women knew that makeup *does* expire but said they never throw it away. Some said they feel guilty about tossing products they spent money on. Others thought, *Oh, I'll use it later!*

Be honest: How much of your makeup is over a year old?

If your answer is "a lot," you're not alone.

Most of us don't use up all our makeup, so we don't see a reason to throw it out. Why would we waste unused product? A 2017 survey from Statista found that 75 percent of consumers between the ages of twenty-five and fifty do not finish all their makeup.[3] The average person owns over forty cosmetic products but only uses five of them daily. If you're like most of my clients, you probably thought using expired makeup was fine. It even sounds like a good idea, since it saves money and avoids waste! But some harmful chemicals in our makeup can become more potent after the expiration date.

Remember what we learned about formaldehyde releasers? To review: they are chemical compounds used as preservatives that slowly release formaldehyde, which is a known carcinogen. Studies have shown that more formaldehyde is released with longer storage time and higher temperature.[4] That's a problem when you consider how long the average person keeps their tube of mascara! As cosmetic products slowly decompose over time, more and more formaldehyde becomes present in the product. This study found that exposure to heat also increased the amount released and that the amount depended on the type of cosmetic too.

Shelf-life guidelines developed and recommended by the cosmetic industry vary, depending on the particular product and how it's used. In general, most cosmetics are formulated and tested for a shelf life of one to three years. However, not all products are required to show expiration dates. It's also true that cosmetics can expire before the expiration date if they are exposed to heat, moisture, or tampering. If you left the lid off your concealer or stored mascara in a cosmetic case in a hot car—or even if a suitcase containing makeup sits on a tarmac on a hot day—it could cause an increase in the amount of formaldehyde released in your makeup.

There are other safety issues with expired makeup too, beyond the harmful chemical exposures. Old makeup can become a breeding ground for bacteria that can lead to possible infection. Mascara can pose a particular risk because of the repeated microbial exposure and the risk of eye infections. If your mascara dries out, never add water—or (worse!) saliva—as that will introduce bacteria to the product. And if you *do* have an eye infection, you definitely need to stop using eye makeup altogether and toss the products you were using when your eye infection began.

How long to keep cosmetics

The FDA considers it to be the manufacturer's responsibility to determine a product's shelf life and states on its website that "there are no U.S. laws or regulations that require cosmetics to have specific shelf lives or have expiration dates on their labels."[5]

A couple of terms to remember:

An **expiration date** is the date after which the product is expired and should not be used anymore.

The **shelf life** of a product means how long you can expect the product to stay safe, maintain its appearance, and perform as expected.

It's pretty easy to tell how long you should use your cosmetics. Just look for the "period after opening" (PAO) symbol on the label

The 12M symbol pictured above means that you can use the product for up to twelve months after opening. If you see this same symbol with a 6M, that means you can use the product for up to six months after opening. A 3M would mean three months, and so on. One way to follow this guideline is to mark the date you opened the product on the bottom near the symbol.

There are several reasons why you want to make sure your products are not expired or used past their PAO or expiration date:

- Preservatives can break down over time, leaving the products vulnerable to fungi and bacteria.
- Products may change color over time.
- Emulsifiers, used to blend oil and water evenly in products, can separate.

Personally, I always recommend tossing products that are close to their expiration date or PAO dates, and don't try to push past it just to make them last a little longer. Why? Mostly because of the increased risk of formaldehyde releasers, as we talked about earlier. The American Academy of Ophthalmology recommends replacing liquid products like mascara and liquid eyeliner about every three months.[6] The same rule applies for items like liquid lipliner. An easy way to remember this is when the season changes, so should your mascara.

MAKEUP EXPIRATION DATE SAFETY

→ Look for the PAO symbol (the jar with the number, followed by M) to know how long a product is good for after opening.

→ Use a marker to mark the product with the date opened near that symbol.

→ Replace cosmetics that are near the expiration date.

→ Store cosmetics away from heat and light.

→ Wash hands before dipping fingers into products.

→ Don't add water to mascara or cosmetics that dry out or harden.

SAFE COSMETIC SHOPPING

→ Look at makeup as a seasonal purchase: buy new makeup to use for fall, winter, spring, and summer.

→ Buy small quantities of cosmetics.

→ At the start of every season, toss out your cosmetics and purchase fresh batches.

SAFE COSMETIC STORAGE

→ Keep cosmetics away from heat and light.

→ Always keep your personal care products in your carry-on luggage.

→ Never leave makeup in your car.

I'll show you how to look for specific expiration dates given by the manufacturer later in this chapter, but there are also some general rules to follow. In Chapters 7 and 8, I gave you some "quick and dirty" tips to follow while shopping for new cosmetic products. Now, I'll give you a more comprehensive list that will show you how to overhaul your cosmetic products all at once, if that's an approach that appeals to you. Remember, the goal is to make small changes that stick over time, so you don't need to do too much too soon. And if you just stick with the small changes we've already covered in this section, you're already doing an amazing job.

Two steps to slightly greener beauty

Step One: Makeup expiration date guidelines

Eyeliner: six months to a year

Mascara: three to six months

Blush, eye shadow, and other powders: one to two years

Foundation: six months to two years

Lipstick: two years

Natural products: three to six months*

*   According to makeup artist Jamie Greenberg, if you store natural products in the fridge, they'll last a little longer.

Step Two: Avoid the following

Fragrance

Methylisothiazolinone

Mineral oil

Parabens

Phthalates

Sodium lauryl sulfate

Triclosan

Formaldehyde releasers (which include DMDM hydantoin, quaternium-15, diazolidinyl urea, and imidazolidinyl urea)

Ethanolamines (DEA, MEA, TEA)

1,4-dioxane (ingredients that end in *-eth*, PEG ingredients, polysorbate 20, 60 and 80)

Stressed about remembering all this the next time you walk into Sephora? Go to slightlygreenerbook.com.

If this sounds overwhelming, use the Slightly Greener Method road map in the Resources section to decide what to prioritize avoiding for your and your family's unique needs, and then work your way up from there.

Slightly greener full cosmetic cleanout

Step 1: Prepare

Grab your skin care products and makeup bag. Place all your products on an easy-to-reach counter for easy sorting. Separate them into four groups:

1. What you use daily
2. What you use frequently (three to four days a week)

3. What you use occasionally (once or twice a month or just on special occasions)

4. What you've had forever and may be expired (we've all got 'em!)

Step 2: Toss expired items

Old cosmetics can be a breeding ground for bacteria, and some toxins can actually increase over time and with exposure to heat and light.

Most shampoo products have a shelf life of up to three years, but when in doubt, throw it out. If the product is old, some of the preservatives in it can be more harmful. If the shampoo bottle has been exposed to heat or light or if it has been sitting on the shelf for too long, toss it.

Tip: I use a Sharpie to mark the date when I open a new bottle of shampoo or conditioner. Also look for the little sign on the back of the bottle that indicates what the shelf life is.

To dispose of makeup properly

If you're throwing away blush or makeup powder, you can put the extra powder into a ziplock bag so that it doesn't spill out and ultimately end up in the soil or in the water, further contaminating the environment with harmful chemicals. Once you've done that, you can throw away the palettes or whatever container it came in. In the future, look for recyclable palettes so that you can be certain that the palettes won't end up in a landfill.

Step 3: Keep everything in the occasional pile

As you go further through the Slightly Greener Method and replace more and more, you can revisit this pile and replace those that have deal-breaking ingredients.

Step 4: Set aside the products you use most often

Replace those that have your deal-breaker ingredients.

Step 5: Replace your most-used products in the daily group

Replace your top two or three most-used items first. The next time you go shopping after that, replace the next one or two most used, and go on from there.

Step 6: Now do the same for your personal care products

This includes items such as shampoo and hair care products, toothpaste, deodorant, body wash, hand soap, shaving cream, etc.

Ingredients to Avoid in Cosmetics and Personal Care Products

INGREDIENT	FOUND IN	HEALTH EFFECTS
Triclosan	Antibacterial products, including dish soap, some school supplies, and hand sanitizer	· Acts as an endocrine disruptor · Linked to increased allergies
Ethanolamines (DEA, MEA, TEA)	Soaps, shampoos, conditioner, baby wash, hand soaps	· Linked to liver tumors · Risk of contamination with nitrosamines (known cancer causers)
Sodium lauryl sulfate	Soaps, shampoos, bubble bath, body wash, facial soap, toothpaste, shaving cream	· Can be contaminated with different carcinogens · Linked to hair loss (in shampoo) · Highly irritating to the skin · May be a cause of canker sores (when in toothpaste)
Mineral oil	Eye shadow, blush, lip gloss, lotions, hair products	· Inhibits skin's oil production · Can prevent the release of toxins through the skin · Possibly contaminated with cancer-causing hydrocarbons
Phthalates	Mascara and nail polish; can hide under the term *fragrance*	· Known as a probable human carcinogen · Act as endocrine disruptors · Linked to lower IQ with prenatal exposure

INGREDIENT	FOUND IN	HEALTH EFFECTS
Fragrance	Hair care, cosmetics, baby wipes, body wash, bubble bath, nail polish, perfumes, body spray, hand sanitizer	• Can be made up of dozens to hundreds of chemicals, including some that act as endocrine disruptors • Linked to cancer and lower IQ • Considered to be a trade secret so individual ingredients are not required to be disclosed
Parabens (methylparaben, propylparaben, butylparaben, and ethylparaben)	Shampoo, deodorant, shave gels, moisturizers, lotions, sunscreens	• Act as endocrine disruptors • Have been found in biopsied breast cancer tumors
Methylisothiazolinone	Shampoos, baby wipes, sunscreens, moisturizers	• Strong allergen • May be toxic to the immune system • May be toxic to the brain and nervous system
Formaldehyde releasers (quaternium-15, diazolidinyl urea, DMDM hydantoin, formalin)	Nail polish, bubble bath, baby wipes, body wash, hair care	• Formaldehyde is a known cancer causer • Linked to organ damage
1,4-dioxane (ingredients that contain PEG, or end in -eth)	Bubble bath, baby wipes, body wash, hair care	• Probable human carcinogen • Toxic to kidneys and nervous system

Part IV

Slightly Greener Cleaning

10

What's Hiding in Cleaning Supplies, Dust, and Indoor Air

The famous American actress and comedienne Phyllis Diller said, "Housework can't kill you, but why take a chance?" I'm with her. My idea of a relaxing Sunday does not include a broom. So trust me: you can follow Diller's less-is-more cleaning ethos and still have a healthy home. Of course housework can't kill you, but minor adjustments to the way you clean *can* make a positive impact on your long-term health and that of your kids. Join me in letting out a big exhale—*Ahhh!* We don't have to become cleaning experts to keep our homes healthy. Just a few small tweaks to the way you are cleaning now will make a huge difference!

The first step is to pay attention to how we clean and what we currently use when doing so. It helps to first be aware of the main ways that toxins emerge in the air of our homes. The key areas to pay attention to are cleaning supplies and products, indoor air quality, and dust. We will go through each one together and learn slightly greener tips for each of these components of healthy home cleaning.

First, let's think about the different cleaning supplies you have in your home. Have you ever counted or even just paused to consider how many of them you own? What about candles and air fresheners, including plug-ins and sprays? Take a quick break from this book and go get them. Be sure to grab them all—check under the kitchen sink, in the laundry room, under bathroom sinks, and in the garage. Gather your cleaning products together in one central location and count them. How many cleaners do you have? No judgment here. I started out with over thirty the first time I did this! Now do the same with your candles and air fresheners. How many did you find?

Don't toss them yet! Put them in an out-of-the-way place for now, although I'm sure you'll want to lose most of them once you see how easy it is to make your own or purchase a safer option. At the end of this section, I'll show you how to dispose of them safely—whether you decide to get rid of just one product, a few, or all of them.

The problem with cleaning supplies

If you're like me, you might have a lot of cleaning products that you're not even using. What's the problem with harmful ingredients if they are under your sink? Well, it turns out that chemicals from cleaning products, candles, scented plug-ins, fabric softener, flooring, and furniture can off-gas into the air. This means that cleaners can emit fumes even while sitting idle in your cabinets, affecting the air quality in your home. The good news is that cleaning products are very easy control. It's so easy to make your own, and many of the ingredients to do so are probably already in your pantry. If you're not the DIY type, don't stress. This isn't the only route to safer cleaning. There are many safer options available for purchase.

The problem with traditional cleaning products is that they often contain harsh chemicals. As we've seen with other types of toxin exposure, this is a problem for our kids, as damage from cleaning products can occur even before birth. Studies have found that prenatal exposure as early as the first trimester can lead to increased lower respiratory infections in babies and children and can continue to lead to respiratory problems later in life. A study in the UK also suggested that children whose mothers frequently use chemical based household products during pregnancy are more likely to wheeze persistently throughout early childhood.[1] Ingredients like MEA (which is found in floor cleaners, laundry detergents, and all-purpose cleaners) and ammonium quaternary compounds (which are typically found in disinfecting sprays and toilet bowl cleaners) have both been shown to induce occupational asthma in cleaning workers. For example, a 2011 study published in the journal *Allergy and Clinical Immunology* reported that janitorial workers have twice the rate of occupational asthma as other workers.[2] In this study, asthma risk was associated with kitchen cleaning, specifically with oven cleaners, as well as furniture polishing.

Another example of cleaning products that can negatively impact health are laundry detergent pods. These easy-to-use alternatives to pouring laundry detergent have only been on the market for seven years. When they first came out, people were excited. Consumers loved the idea of just tossing that little pod into the washer—no measuring, no slimy spills. Plus those pods were an inspiring innovation that promised to make cleaning just a little bit easier. What was not to love? But between 2012 and 2017, laundry detergent pods have resulted in over seventy thousand calls to poison control centers.[3] While the pods looked harmless at first, children accidentally ingested the contents and occasionally squirted it in their eyes or spilled it on their skin. Children and the elderly are especially susceptible to the dangers of detergent pods, due to the potentially lethal combination of toxins and candy-like packaging. According to *CBS New York*, eight deaths to date have been associated with ingesting the packets: two infant children and six adults with a history of dementia.[4]

After hearing that, you might be wondering: What can we do? And there's excellent news, because the answer is that there's *a lot* we can do. Applying the Slightly Greener Method to cleaning is one of my favorite topics to talk about, because there are so many easy options for cleaning. While it's tempting to have a different cleaner for just about everything in the house—multipurpose cleaners, glass cleaners, toilet cleaners, and so on—it's easy to make simple DIY products that can clean most things in your house.

How do you know if your home is toxic?

If you're concerned that your home might have an unhealthy amount of environmental toxins in it, there are a few different ways that you can make an assessment. Do you have a family member in your home who gets sick often? What about allergies and asthma? While these can be caused by a variety of sources, some of which are unavoidable, they can also be an indication that the toxin level in your home is unhealthy. Many cleaning chemicals are linked to allergies and asthma. Have you or anyone you live with noticed that you feel healthier outside your home? That can also be a sign. If your allergy or asthma symptoms ease up or if other symptoms—like headaches, for instance—go away when you're out of the house, this can be a sign that the toxin level in your home could be worth looking into.

The importance of our indoor environment

Even if you're not experiencing symptoms like headaches or allergies, it's important to remember that environmental toxins in our home are harmful to *all* of us. Even if you're not feeling the effects of exposure to harmful chemicals immediately, we don't know the effects of long-term exposure. You might not think that just sitting inside your home and breathing the air could be toxic. But as always I say, don't freak out. There's a Slightly Greener Method for solving this too. In this chapter, you will learn about harmful chemicals hiding in cleaning supplies, in the dust collecting in the corners of your home, and even in the indoor air you breathe. Are you with me? Let's dive in.

We need to pay close attention to the quality of our indoor environment because people who live in the United States spend more than 90 percent of their time indoors.[5] For most of the day, Americans are holed up in their homes, workplaces, schools, gyms, or cars. Most of these places are full of dust and other things that can be harmful to our health. We also use cleaning products that contain endocrine disruptors and chemicals that are toxic to the brain, respiratory system, and reproductive system, among other undesirable health effects.

What is most important here—just as it was with food and cosmetics—is figuring out which small changes we can make that will be the most impactful. Harmful chemicals in cleaning supplies, in indoor air, and in dust are more potent for children, but so are the positive effects from removing them; reducing the amount of harmful chemicals in kids' environments can have a significant impact on their health. Kids come into direct contact with indoor dust; they crawl around and pick up dust off the ground in their fingers, put their hands into their mouths, and generally just spend more time on the ground around dust than adults do. So what exactly are they picking up with those cute little hands?

Common toxins in dust

By now, you know that dust can hold toxins that can make us sick. Here are a few of the most common chemicals found in dust (that you will now avoid by dusting your high traffic areas just a bit more):

TOXIN	FOUND IN	HEALTH CONCERNS
Phthalates	Vinyl flooring, vinyl shower curtains/shower curtain liners, and soft rubber toys; hides in fragrances (in personal care/beauty and cleaning products, etc.)	• Linked to developmental issues, hormone disruption, reproduction and fertility issues • Found to lower IQ in children born to mothers who had the highest levels when tested
Flame retardants	Furniture with polyurethane foam, electronics, some brands of high chairs, mattresses, car seats, and some children's pajamas	• Cancer causing • Linked to reproductive/ fertility and nervous system issues, obesity, hormone disruption, thyroid issues, and behavior and attention issues in children
Fluorinated chemicals	Nonstick cookware, stain- and water-resistant clothing and furniture, lining of fast food wrappers, and lining of microwave popcorn bags	• Linked to cancer, immune system problems, developmental issues, low birth rates, and infertility
Lead	Paint (in homes built before 1978), cosmetics, art supplies, air, water, soil, and certain careers and industry (lead can be brought into the home from those exposed at work)	• Neurological effects and lower IQ • Although lead exposure over time can affect adults, kids are more susceptible to lead exposure

Once you've implemented a tiny bit of extra dusting, there are some other practical ways you can reduce the dust buildup in your home. Add one tip at a time until these changes become habits. The first tip is to remove your shoes when you enter your home. We not only bring dirt inside on our shoes but dust too. Once you've made that change, I recommend you ramp up (to a slightly greener degree) vacuuming as well as damp dusting and mopping the areas where you—or your kids—spend the most time. Dusting and mopping with a damp towel is effective because the moisture will lift up the dust rather than pushing it around. Next, I suggest you wash your hands more frequently with warm water and soap. Finally, buying safer products for your home will reduce the amount of harmful chemicals you're exposed to in the first place, and fewer toxins will wind up in your household dust.

SEVEN TIPS TO LOWER YOUR EXPOSURE TO DUST

1. Don't stress about dusting every room every day. Concentrate on places where your family spends the most time, such as bedrooms and floors/play areas where your children hang out.

2. Take your shoes off before entering your home. You'd be surprised what comes in on shoes!

3. Damp mop rather than sweep. Sweeping just moves the dust around.

4. Damp dust rather than dry dusting with a Swiffer or feather duster; this also moves dust around. Dust with a safe dusting spray or use a DIY dusting spray (using toxic chemicals just adds to the problem).

5. Vacuum frequently, and use a vacuum with a HEPA filter.

6. Wash hands with soap and water frequently, especially before eating. (Hand sanitizer doesn't count!)

7. Buy safer products as often as possible to cut down on overall toxins in your home.

Indoor air quality

Do you know what the EPA has called the nation's number one environmental health problem? Indoor air pollution. We often assume it's safe, but the air inside our homes and offices can be two to five times—and occasionally more than one hundred times—more polluted than outdoor air.[6] Have you ever heard of sick building syndrome? Sick building syndrome is a condition that can cause headaches, fatigue, difficulty concentrating, nausea, dizziness and irritated throats, nasal passages, and eyes when someone is confined to an enclosed building, like an office, with contaminated air.[7] In 2016, researchers at Harvard, Syracuse, and SUNY Upstate Medical universities examined twenty-four people in four different atmospheres to determine how the air quality of a workspace might affect cognitive function.[8] The researchers set up the four different environments to see which provided the best (and worst) air quality. These environments were intended to match the air found in three different building conditions: a conventional office building, a "green" office building with low VOC concentrations, a "green" office building with low VOC concentrations plus enhanced ventilation, and conditions with artificially elevated levels of CO_2, independent of ventilation. VOCs (volatile organic compounds) are compounds that easily become vapors or gas. They are released from consumer products like solvents, paint, glue, barbecues, burning candles, stoves, glass cleaners, and dishwashing or laundry detergents.

The scientists gave everyone the same cognitive functioning test that measured nine different cognitive functioning parameters, such as

information usage, strategy, and crisis response, and—no surprise—
the worst results came from the conventional building. Scores were
61 percent higher in the green building and a remarkable 101 percent
better in the green building with enhanced ventilation, implying that
the quality of indoor air can not only affect physical health but mental
functioning too. Researchers attributed the higher scores in the green
buildings to fewer VOCs and less carbon dioxide in the atmosphere.

Indoor air pollution is caused partly by building materials but
also by chemicals from cleaning products, candles, plug-ins, fabric
softeners, flooring, and furniture releasing fumes that affect air
quality. Poor indoor air quality has become a bigger problem in the
last couple of decades, with an increased focus on building energy-
efficient homes. While employing a home design that saves energy
sounds great in theory, these homes are often sealed up tighter, without adequate air exchange to clear toxins off-gassing from the products in the house. Your heating and cooling bills might see the benefit,
but air quality and health can suffer.

To keep your home smelling good, do you ever use products that
promise to "freshen" the air? How about scented candles or lemony
fresh cleaning products? I once did too. But if you think about it, it
makes sense that some of these products are harmful. (Spoiler alert:
they're not made with real lemons.)

"What? Even candles can be bad for you?" some of my clients
say. They are often very surprised to learn that a simple candle on
your dinner table can be toxic. The truth is that any product with
artificial fragrance can release toxins and chemicals into the air you

breathe at home. After my client Susan stopped using plug-in fresheners and replaced her conventional scented candles with soy-based alternatives, both she and her son reported having fewer irritated, sore throats. Toni in South Carolina had a three-year-old daughter with sleep issues and allergies. When we started working together, she mentioned that her daughter's congestion and sleep challenges were her most pressing health issues, so we started by taking a couple of ingredients out of her child's diet. After that, we removed artificial fragrances in her home and made some DIY cleaning products that don't have negative effects on the respiratory system. Now her daughter has fewer stuffy noses and also sleeps great most nights.

Surprisingly, health risks from polluted indoor air can be more harmful than outdoor air pollution, which is a problem considering that 90 percent of the population spends their time indoors.[9] The average home contains five hundred to fifteen hundred toxic chemicals, and the majority of these chemicals are not required to be listed on product labels. While some of these chemicals may be OK in small doses, we don't know what happens when they combine, as many of them have never been tested individually, let alone in combination with other chemicals. The EPA only requires companies to list active disinfecting ingredients and "chemicals of known concern" on their labels.[10] The big loophole here, of course, is the word *known*. Safety testing isn't required by the companies or the EPA or even by the Consumer Product Safety Commission. The companies that manufacture traditional cleaning products argue against disclosure for competition reasons, saying they want to keep their formulations proprietary.

Quick tips for safer indoor air

The first thing I recommend you do is stop using plug-in or aerosol air fresheners to scent the air in your home. Air fresheners don't really "freshen" the air; they simply mask odors and, in the process, let off toxic chemicals. But there are easy ways to freshen the air in your home naturally. First, try to open windows as often as possible to let in fresh air. I also recommend running a fan to circulate air, or try to identify and remove the cause of the smell you're trying to get rid of.

Essential oils are also a great way to keep your house smelling fresh without the harmful effects of conventional air fresheners. You can purchase a diffuser, which is a little device that will break down the oils into smaller molecules and spray them into the air. If you purchase a diffuser, check for details on how many square feet it will cover. Experiment with different combinations of scents. I find that lemon, lavender, and peppermint go great together and can also help with allergy symptoms. Some oils can kill airborne germs too. If you have pets, just be sure to research whether the essential oils are safe for animals, as not all essential oils are pet friendly. I also suggest you toss any scented candles. If you can't bear to part with them, only burn them on special occasions or when company comes over. (Even better if you can burn soy or beeswax candles with lead-free wicks!)

It's also easy to use baking soda to freshen small spaces such as closets, bathrooms, and the fridge. Place a box of open baking soda in these areas, or you can also place a mason jar or container in a room with a half cup of baking soda and a few drops of essential oil to absorb the odor and freshen the room. Get a small mason jar and poke holes in the lid, then pour baking soda into the jar. To make it more decorative, I like to buy a pretty fabric material and poke holes in that as well. Then I pull the fabric tight over the mason jar before screwing on the outer lid around it. You can scent the baking soda by pouring a few drops of essential oils into the blend. Every week or so, just shake the mason jar to release a little more of the scent. This is a great option for bathrooms or other small spaces where you just want a little extra freshening.

When you need more intense freshening, like to keep odors at bay, sprinkle baking soda on carpets, let it sit for a few hours, and vacuum it up. You'll be amazed at how effective this is. The baking soda will absorb the odors from your carpets, just as it does in the refrigerator.

SAFE DISPOSAL OF AEROSOL SPRAYS

Aerosol sprays should be disposed of safely! If the aerosol can is not empty, it is considered hazardous waste. Find out where the nearest waste disposal site is near you.

I also recommend salt lamps. You know how when you're near the ocean or in the mountains, you can literally feel the difference in the fresh air as you breathe it in? When you inhale in those environments, you instantly feel better. You can recreate that experience with a salt lamp. A salt lamp is a chunk of Himalayan salt crystal with the inside hollowed out to make space for a light bulb. When the light is turned on, the salt heats up and releases negative ions, which are typically found in ocean shores, waterfalls, and during storms.[11] These negative ions can bind with indoor air pollutants and make them heavier, caus-ing them to fall to the ground where they are less likely to be inhaled. Indoor air is often very low in negative ions, especially around com-puters and other electronics, so an office is a great place to put a salt lamp.[12] This is one of my favorite ways to purify the air; they are also beautiful when lit and will boost your mood! Salt is hygroscopic by nature, meaning it is able to attract water.[13] The small amount of water vapor in air can contain contaminants such as mold, bacteria, allergens, bacteria, and viruses.[14] The heat from the light bulb inside causes the water to evaporate quickly, which is why most Himalayan salt lamp companies recommended keeping the salt lamp on a plate to prevent the sweating that may occur, especially in high-humidity environments.[15] Bonus: they also may have anxiety- and depression-relieving qualities.[16]

QUICK TIPS FOR HEALTHIER INDOOR AIR

→ Don't use scented plug-ins, spray air fresheners, or candles.

→ Diffuse essential oils to freshen and purify the air.

→ Freshen small spaces with baking soda.

→ Vacuum and mop frequently.

→ Use a salt lamp to purify the air and reduce allergens.

→ Open the windows.

→ Use houseplants.

Ditch the sprays

In addition to the dangers that conventional cleaning products pose, aerosol sprays present unique risks. They are comprised of toxic chemicals and also typically contain ingredients such as hexane and xylene. These ingredients and others like them are not only flammable but can also cause nerve damage and even brain toxicity. Think about what happens when you spray aerosol: the particles are tiny and can enter the bloodstream rapidly when inhaled. Usually, you don't even realize you're inhaling them because they are essentially invisible. But breathing them in can lead to potential health issues. In fact, homes where aerosol sprays and air fresheners are frequently used reported that the mothers had 25 percent more headaches and were 19 percent more likely to suffer from depression.[17] That same study found that infants under six months of age had 30 percent more ear infections and a 22 percent increase in diarrhea compared to those from families using non-spray cleaners.

Cleaning products and kids

Just like the other dangerous chemicals we've discussed throughout the book, cleaning products can be especially harmful to children. Whether or not kids are helping clean, they're often exposed to harsh cleaners in the home. Plus, many of them like to help (before a certain age, of course!). Anyone who is around when someone is cleaning can inhale vapors from the products, which can cause lung damage. And even low levels of exposure to some cleaning chemicals over a lifetime may increase the risk of serious health issues, such as cancer or reproductive issues. Those are some pretty big reasons why I made immediate changes to the household cleaners in our home and also came up with the tips and tricks that I share in this book as well as DIY recipes.

Deadly fumes from oven cleaning?

It's not just the vapors from cleaning products that can cause toxin exposure while cleaning. One of the biggest contributors, believe it or not, is actually your oven. Have you ever used the self-cleaning feature and maybe felt a little nauseous afterward? Or had to cough when you entered the kitchen? Something similar happened to a twenty-nine-year old man in Japan. He fell asleep while boiling water, and when the water evaporated, the pan began to burn. He awoke when the room filled with smoke. Trying to stop the smoke, he put the pan under the sink, and when water hit the pan, a vapor rose up, and he inhaled. A few hours later, he showed up at an emergency room with a fever, labored breathing, and a cough. The man had a rare disease called polymer fume fever that the doctors were able to diagnose quickly because he had brought the pan with him to the emergency room. It had been coated in polytetrafluoroethylene, also known by its brand name, Teflon. This nonstick coating can decompose rapidly under high heat, and when mixed with water, it releases a poisonous vapor. That's exactly how the Japanese man ended up inhaling deadly fumes.[18] Though cases like this are rare, a similar process occurs when we use a self-cleaning oven. Self-cleaning ovens have a Teflon-like, nonstick coating inside. During the self-cleaning cycle, the oven can heat to over 600°F, and this releases toxic fumes into the air. Breathing in these fumes can lead to flu-like symptoms, cough, sore throat, and even breathing difficulties. If there is spilled food in the oven, that is burned during the self-cleaning process, it produces carbon monoxide fumes that can escape through the oven's vents.[19] I hope I've convinced you *never* to hit that Clean Oven button again. However, if you absolutely have to use the self-cleaning feature on your oven, be sure to open all the windows and leave the house while it's working.

Slightly greener cleaning

You likely don't need to toss all your cleaning products out. Let's start small and just look at the products under your sink or wherever you keep your cleaning supplies.

Step 1: Get rid of any product that lists artificial ingredients like glycol ethers (including 2-butoxyethanol), dyes, and fragrances. (Byebye, Windex!)

Step 2: Toss anything that contains propane or isobutane or kerosene or "petroleum gases."[20] These compounds are all derived from petroleum and are more similar to the gasoline you put in your car than anything you would want in your home. I'm also not a fan of the corrosive seminatural products our grandmothers used, including bleach and ammonia. Both have been shown to cause respiratory issues and can be harmful if accidentally spilled on your skin or swallowed.

Ingredients to Avoid in Cleaning Products

INGREDIENT	FOUND IN	HEALTH EFFECTS
Glycol ethers (most common type is 2-butoxyethanol)	Grease cutters and window cleaners (Simple Green, Formula 409, Windex, etc.)	· Liver cancer in lab animals · Exposure by inhalation and skin · Can go through rubber gloves
Alkylphenol ethoxylates (nonylphenol and octylphenol; nonoxynol)	Laundry detergents (may see them listed as "nonionic surfactants"), cleaning products, paint, hair care products, pesticides	· Mimics estrogen · Shown to multiply breast cancer cells in lab tests · May disrupt immune system · Bioaccumulates
Dye	All-purpose cleaners, window cleaners, toilet bowl cleaners, laundry detergents	· Term used to hide chemical info; not sure what ingredients it contains
Ethanolamines (DEA, MEA, TEA)	Degreasing formulas (Fantastik, Formula 409, Easy-Off, etc.), laundry detergents	· Possible contamination with nitrosamines (carcinogens) · Can trigger asthma attacks, even in those without asthma
Fragrance	Multipurpose cleaners, floor cleaners, laundry detergents, dryer sheets, window cleaners, dish soap, dusting sprays	· Endocrine disruption · Can be made up of hundreds, if not thousands of chemicals
Quaternary ammonium compounds (benzalkonium chloride)	Disinfecting sprays (Pine-Sol, Fantastik), fabric softeners and laundry detergents (Purex brand), oven cleaners, drain clog removers	· Can cause asthma and allergic reactions · Can cause severe skin burns and eye damage
Synthetic musk	Soap, cosmetics, laundry detergents, dryer sheets	· Enhances the effects of other toxic chemicals in products · Bioaccumulates

INGREDIENT	FOUND IN	HEALTH EFFECTS
Chlorinated phenol	Toilet bowl cleaners	· Toxic to the respiratory system
Diethylene glycol	Window cleaners	· Depresses the nervous system
Butyl cellusolve	All-purpose and window cleaners	· May damage liver, kidneys, bone marrow, and nervous system
Bleach	Products labeled "with bleach," chlorine bleach, countertop sprays, toilet bowl cleaners	· Can cause irritation in the eyes, mouth, lungs, and skin · Can be fatal if swallowed · Is corrosive internally and externally
Ammonia	Window cleaners, metal polishers, stainless steel and brass polishes, some all-purpose cleaners (especially those labeled "tough on grease")	· Moderate risk for respiratory concerns · Can cause dangerous, even deadly fumes, especially when mixed with bleach products

When in Doubt, Do It Yourself

While it sounds like it could be a daunting process, replacing traditional cleaning products with homemade ones is actually quite simple. When I first started this journey to create a slightly greener home, I had a slew of cleaning products under my kitchen sink. In fact, I owned a different cleaner for each type of surface—counters, glass, toilets, rugs, showers, you name it. It dawned on me that I'd been conditioned to believe that I needed a different cleaner for each material or object in my home. But that was far from the truth, and once again, clever marketing was to blame.

I was initially nervous about substituting homemade versions of cleaning supplies for my old commercial standbys; DIY just wasn't my thing. But once I realized how easy it was to make a homemade toilet bowl cleaner, my attitude quickly shifted. Compared to schlepping to the store, spending a ton of money, and using products that are harmful to your heath, making most products yourself for pennies on the dollar doesn't sound so bad. And I promise you: it's nothing like a complicated recipe that involves hours of preparation or cleanup. It's literally as simple as throwing a couple of things together in a bowl and mixing them together. Your kids could do it. (And they should!)

As I continued to dig up research about the dangers in the conventional cleaning products, I became ever more committed to the process of making my own. Honestly, it became a no-brainer. One study from the National Institutes of Health found that 1,4-dichlorobenzene (or 1,4-DCB), a chemical in air fresheners, toilet deodorizers, and mothballs—found in the blood of 96 percent of Americans!—can cause harm to the lungs.[1] 1,4-DCB is linked to poor lung function and may also contribute to heart disease, stroke, lung cancer, and general morbidity.[2] And as we learned in the last chapter, you—and your kids—might be breathing in harmful chemicals like these without even realizing it.

Toilet bowl cleaners also tend to contain another harmful chemical called hydrochloric acid. This chemical causes eye irritation, kidney damage, and irritation to the respiratory system if breathed in. It's also corrosive to skin. It's not uncommon for pets to drink water out of the toilet. When pets ingest the chemicals from toilet bowl cleaners, it can make them quite ill. In this chapter, I will share my favorite recipes for a DIY toilet bowl cleaner and room freshener that will smell great and can be used repeatedly without any worry of harm. Homemade cleaning products are not only cheaper—and most of the time safer—but they can even be fun to make. If you have kids who like to help, then you can feel better about giving them chores to clean stuff around the house too.

The ingredients in my DIY products are completely safe for kids to be around or use themselves. This is important, because as you will recall, their bodies are more vulnerable to toxic cleaners. They still need to be supervised, of course, but if they like to help you clean, you can feel better knowing they will not be exposed to toxic chemicals. In my opinion, that's an even bigger benefit than the cost savings! My kids are older now, so it's a bit more challenging to employ their help than it was back when they were eager toddlers. But once kids come around to helping with the family chores, they usually get a sense of pride and accomplishment from helping out and contributing to the family's health and well-being. And I rest easier at night knowing that I've created a healthier home with fewer toxic chemicals that are releasing harmful fumes into the air.

Baking soda and vinegar for DIY recipes

Baking soda and vinegar are staples in my house. I always have several containers of each on hand. Just these two ingredients can be used for so many DIY recipes. You really don't need specialized cleaners for each area of your house, and you definitely don't need harsh cleaners. Many DIY recipes call for mixing the ingredients and keeping them in a glass spray bottle. But when you're using baking soda and vinegar, these are two that you don't want to mix ahead of time—they will fizz and make a mess everywhere if stored combined together. Before you start making DIY cleaners, make sure you have a decent amount of both ingredients on hand. Unlike air fresheners, which just cover up odors, baking soda actually absorbs the odors that can cause kitchens, bathrooms, and other areas in your home to smell bad. The reason? Most odors are acidic, and since baking soda is basic, it causes a chemical reaction to neutralize them. This acid/base reaction is also what makes the baking soda/vinegar combination so powerful. In some instances, baking soda can also work better than everyday soap. While both soap and baking soda are basic, soap is made up of fat molecules, which can make it less harsh. But baking soda *is* harsh and has a more abrasive effect on the stains and dirt, allowing it to lift dirt off surfaces.[3]

TWO DIY CLEANING PRODUCTS TO KEEP IN STOCK

Baking soda and white vinegar. You can clean most things in your home with these two simple and safe ingredients!

Here are my favorite cleaners to make at home. All of them are surprisingly easy to make. Even if you *just* make your own window cleaner and toilet bowl cleaner, you'll lower the overall exposure in your home and save nearly $100 a year (or more).[4] *Please note in all the DIY cleaners that use water, I recommend distilled water so it doesn't leave streaks or mineral deposits behind.

Getting started with DIY cleaning products

While you may not need every item on this list, here are some helpful ingredients to have on hand to make your own DIY cleaning recipes:

- ▸ Baking soda
- ▸ Hydrogen peroxide (3%)
- ▸ White vinegar
- ▸ Castile soap
- ▸ Distilled water
- ▸ Essential oils (optional)
- ▸ Glass spray bottles
- ▸ Cellulose sponge

SLIGHTLY GREENER CLEANING TIP

To save money on buying glass spray bottles, buy vinegar in glass bottles and reuse them to make your DIY window cleaner and all-purpose spray. Pump sprays from old cleaning products fit on these bottles. Simply screw them on the top, and you're set!

Here are some of my favorite DIY cleaners for you to try. And remember, if you don't have time or if DIY isn't your thing, check the Resources section for safer brands you can buy.

Oven cleaner

Why you should avoid it: Products such as oven cleaners are full of harmful ingredients, such as lye (caustic soda), ethylene glycol, and methylene chloride. These ingredients are linked to asthma, other respiratory problems, and possibly cancer. Oven cleaners also commonly contain glycol ethers, which are probable human carcinogens and have been shown to damage red blood cells, and recent studies have linked prenatal exposure to cognitive impairment in children.

How to DIY: First, remove the oven racks (it's a great time to clean these now too!), then wipe out all the crumbs and charred food remnants. You should do this regularly—even when you're not doing a deep oven clean—as we now know that the charred food remnants sitting on the bottom of your oven can actually give off toxic fumes when reheated. Sprinkle a thin layer of baking soda across the bottom of the oven. Next, spray vinegar onto the baking soda layer and watch as it begins to bubble and fizz and start lifting up the grease and stains. You may have to repeat this a couple of times to get everything out—especially the first time you do it—but it works really well. If you have trouble getting all the baking soda out, just repeat spraying it with the vinegar, and it comes right up! For extra tough stains, pour water into a baking dish and heat the water in the oven, letting the steam loosen grime, and then do the baking soda and vinegar combination.

Toilet bowl cleaner

Why you should avoid it: Traditional toilet bowl cleaners can contain harmful chemicals such as sodium hypochlorite (linked to developmental and reproductive effects, vision damage, and nervous system and digestive effects) and sodium hydroxide (which can cause respiratory effects and damage to vision). Some also contain hydrochloric acid, which is corrosive to the eyes, skin, and mucous membranes.

How to DIY: There are two options I like to use:

1. **Overnight toilet bowl cleaner:** Pour half a 32-ounce bottle of white vinegar into the toilet bowl before bed, then scrub it in the morning.

2. **Quick clean:** Pour some vinegar into the toilet bowl and then baking soda right after. After it fizzes, I scrub the toilet. You can also add some essential oils for extra scent and cleaning if you want, but it's not necessary. I like to use lemon essential oil for freshening or tea tree essential oil for a little extra cleaning boost.

Carpet stain remover

Why you should avoid it: Like many cleaning products, it's hard to tell what the exact ingredients of a carpet stain remover are. Many of them don't state any specific ingredients, and others say very vague terms, such as "enzymes." But which enzymes? And do they have negative health effects? Many carpet stain removers also use solvents that are similar to dry cleaning chemicals so they can lift off dirt and grease without having to use water. Acute inhalation exposure to these chemicals can cause upper respiratory tract irritation and kidney issues as well as neurological effects, including headaches, dizziness, and behavioral changes. Carpet stain removers often contain perchloroethylene, also known as perc, which is a colorless, sweet-smelling liquid also commonly used in dry cleaning and stain removers. The International Agency for Research on Cancer has classified perchloroethylene as a probable cancer causer in humans.

How to DIY: Guess what I use to clean carpets? Yep, I get a lot of mileage out of that baking soda and vinegar solution; it's my go-to carpet stain remover too. (It has even gotten red wine and elderberry syrup out of my carpet!) Just as I do with the toilet bowl cleaner, I eyeball the amount I need to use. Be sure to spot test an out-of-the-way area first. Sprinkle a very thin layer of baking soda over the stain, and then spray vinegar over it and let it fizz. You can see the stain actually lifting out of the carpet. Blot it—don't rub—with a light-colored towel or cloth. You may need to repeat more than once to get the stain out, but it works insanely well.

QUICK DIY CLEANING TIPS

→ Keep baking soda and vinegar in each bathroom cabinet and under the kitchen sink (I buy the gallon-size for bathrooms).

→ For the oven cleaner and stain remover, buy vinegar in glass bottles.

→ An easy way to recycle some of your not-as-safe cleaning products is to save the spray pumps, wash them out well, and attach them to the glass vinegar bottles for an easy spray bottle. When the vinegar solution runs low, refill from a gallon size container of vinegar.

Window cleaner

Why you should avoid it: Window cleaners, like Windex, typically contain fragrance, which we know can be made up of dozens of different chemicals. They sometimes also contain glycol ether, depending on the brand, which can aggravate asthma, is linked to fertility issues, and can damage red blood cells. Sodium laureth sulfate is another ingredient you may see, which is linked to the probable cancer causer 1,4-dioxane. Ethanolamines such as MEA are also common and can be contaminated with cancer-causing nitrosamines.

How to DIY: For a safer window cleaner, I use a 50/50 solution of white vinegar and distilled water and find it's just as effective as traditional window cleaning products. The first time you use this solution on your windows, you may see streaks, but don't be alarmed or think it's not working. Conventional window cleaners can leave a wax film buildup behind. To get rid of this, just spray the glass with rubbing alcohol and wipe down. You can also add just a couple of drops of lemon essential oil to the vinegar and distilled water solution for a clean scent.

IMPORTANT!

Do NOT mix these ingredients together, because they can create harmful gases:

Bleach and ammonia

Bleach and vinegar

Bleach and rubbing alcohol

Vinegar and hydrogen peroxide

Be extra careful when using your DIY products if you're also using regular cleaners in the same area (for example, using a DIY window cleaner with a regular toilet bowl cleaner in the same bathroom).

Mold and mildew remover

Why you should avoid it: These cleaners typically contain the corrosive ingredients chlorine and alkyl ammonium chlorides, which are known to cause breathing problems as well as eye, throat, and skin irritation. And believe it or not, vinegar works better than bleach for cleaning up mold! Bleach can brighten up the area and kill the mold on the surface, but it doesn't get to the roots of the mold. White vinegar kills about 82 percent of mold and can penetrate porous surfaces to kill the roots.

How to DIY: Pour white vinegar into a spray bottle. Then thoroughly spray the surface and let it sit for an hour. Follow by rinsing the area with a warm, damp cloth (do not soak the area with water). If the area needs scrubbing, you can make a paste of baking soda and water in a bowl and scrub with a sponge.

Air freshener

Why you should avoid it: Air fresheners, as we now know, are a misleading name. Rather than freshening the air, they actually fill it with chemicals that cover *up* smells. So the air isn't really fresh at all but instead filled with both odors and chemicals. Many air fresheners also contain fragrance, that mysterious combination of unknown chemicals.

How to DIY: Diffusing essential oils is a great way to help purify the air and keep your house smelling fresh without the harmful effects of plug-in and spray air fresheners or heavily scented candles. When buying diffusers, look at how many square feet they cover, and place them in the areas of your home that need them most. There are also several studies published in medical journals on the health benefits of essential oils; they have been touted as a way to improve sleep, lessen anxiety, and reduce headaches.[5] If you have pets, please do research before you diffuse oils, as certain oils may not be recommended for them.

Furniture polish

Why you should avoid it: Furniture polish commonly contains phenols, which can cause respiratory problems and damage to the cardiovascular and nervous system, and nitrobenzene, which is easily absorbed through the skin, is extremely toxic, and is a probable human carcinogen.

How to DIY: Mix the following ingredients in a glass bottle

3/4 cup olive oil

1/4 cup distilled vinegar

1 teaspoon lemon juice

Approximately 40 drops lemon or orange essential oil

Test in a hidden spot first before using on a new piece of furniture, and be sure to wipe it off well.

FOUR EASY WAYS TO FRESHEN INDOOR AIR

1. **Don't use air fresheners or candles.** These only mask odors and let toxic chemicals into the air. Open windows, run a fan to circulate air, and also try to identify and remove the cause of the smell.

2. **Diffuse essential oils.** Essential oils are a great way to help purify the air and keep your house smelling fresh without the harmful effects of conventional air fresheners. Check the diffuser for how many square feet it will cover, and place it where it is needed most. Experiment with different combinations, such as lemon, lavender, and peppermint. Some oils can kill airborne germs, so they not only smell great but can help keep you healthy as well.

3. **Keep baking soda in the fridge** (and where the dog sleeps!) Place a mason jar or container with half a cup of baking soda and a few drops of essential oil in a room to absorb the odor and freshen the room. You can also sprinkle baking soda at the bottom of wastebaskets and trash cans to absorb odors.

4. **Sweep or vacuum a lot**. This will help remove dust, which is a huge source of household toxins.

When DIY isn't the best option

Of course, there will be times when you choose not to DIY. Perhaps you're out of baking soda or vinegar or just don't have the time. And for some cleaning products—like laundry detergent and all-purpose cleaners—I find that the safer brand options are preferable to DIY. I would love to make my laundry detergent, but I simply haven't come across a recipe I like. Instead, I use a safer brand for washing laundry and wool balls to replace dryer sheets as a fabric softener. For all-purpose cleaning around the house, I also use electrolyzed water instead of creating my own DIY cleaning solution. Electrolyzed water is water that has been converted into hypochlorous acid and sodium hydroxide to create a nontoxic cleaner and disinfectant. It's included on the EPA's list of disinfectants.[6] Look in the Resources section for the brands I recommend.

Eliminate bacteria and viruses

Occasionally, you may want to do a serious disinfecting of your home. Good news! You can get your house just as clean and germ-free with safe DIY products as you can with Lysol and bleach. Perhaps you have a sick family member or someone who is immune compromised coming to visit. In those cases, I will share with you what I do for my own home.

Bacteria are living organisms. We have trillions of them in our bodies, and most of them keep us healthy by aiding important functions like digestion. But about 1 percent of bacteria can cause illnesses, like upper respiratory infections, pneumonia, and food poisoning. Viruses, on the other hand, aren't live organisms—they need a host cell to reproduce. But like bacteria, they spread when they come into contact with the host. The good news is that many bacteria and viruses are killed with proper hand washing hygiene and regular surface area cleaning. Cleaning your home using these tips will get rid of bacteria and viruses.

1. **Wash hands with plain soap and water.** Believe it or not, washing your hands with regular soap and water is *the best* defense against bacteria and viruses that can make us ill. Why? Because some infectious viruses are what's called an "envelope" protein, which is somewhat easy to break down. The fatty components of soap help to break down the fatty lipids in the outer covering of the virus.

   How to do it: Wash your hands for at least twenty seconds.

That ensures the soap is foaming up and your hands are creating enough friction to destroy the virus's protective coating.

2. **Use hand sanitizer correctly.** When handwashing isn't an option, use hand sanitizer. If you're out and about and don't have access to soap and water, this is a good alternative.

   How to do it: Spray or pour a generous amount on your hands, making sure to cover palms and fingertips, and rub hands together until dry. It's best to wash hands first if possible because the sanitizer works best on clean, nongreasy hands.

3. **Clean dirty surfaces first before disinfecting.** Dirt and grime can reduce the effectiveness of the disinfectant.

   How to do it: Clean surfaces first with an all-purpose cleaner or plain soap and water (with some good elbow grease behind it, especially on surfaces like countertops), and then disinfect.

4. **Disinfect surfaces.** Some harmful bacteria, such as certain common flu and cold viruses, are relatively easy to kill, so there are simple things around your home that will work to disinfect.

   How to do it: After cleaning, use one of the following to disinfect:

   a. Hydrogen peroxide: Look for 3% on the label, which indicates household peroxide, as opposed to hair bleach or food grade hydrogen peroxide, which has a higher concentration. After cleaning the surface, spray hydrogen peroxide on and let sit for at least ten minutes before wiping away. Don't use on fabrics, as it can discolor certain materials.

   b. Rubbing alcohol: Use at least 70 percent concentration, and let sit for a minute or two. Note that this can discolor some plastics and can damage some finishes on wooden furniture, so always use it in an inconspicuous spot first to make sure no discoloration will occur.

c. Electrolyzed water: This is tap water that has been converted into hypochlorous acid and sodium hydroxide, making it a nontoxic cleaner and disinfectant.

5. **Disinfect high-touch areas several times a day.** This includes doorknobs and handles, faucets, sinks, tables, light switches, cabinet and drawer handles, refrigerator handles, countertops, remote controls, cell phones, tablets, etc.

How to do it: First, make sure surfaces are clean and not visibly dirty. If using hydrogen peroxide or rubbing alcohol, pour them into a spray bottle. Spray onto surfaces and let the disinfectant sit (always use in an inconspicuous spot first to make sure no discoloration will occur). A product that is labeled "disinfectant" means that product claims to destroy the bacteria and viruses noted on the label.[7]

Viruses such as the flu, measles, or the common cold live longest on hard surfaces (like steel and plastic), whereas bacteria (such as the one that causes strep throat or *E. coli*) tend to live longer on porous materials.[8] In general, bacteria remain infectious longer than viruses. Some viruses like the common cold can survive on indoor surfaces for several days but usually don't cause infections after twenty-four hours.[9] Similarly, some bacteria live for only for a short while, like *E. coli*, which only lives for hours outside the body, while others, like anthrax, can live for decades! The best thing you can do is wipe down high-touch areas frequently, especially in winter or if someone in your home is ill.

6. **Use heat**. According to the World Health Organization, temperatures of 140°F to 150°F are enough to kill most viruses and bacteria.[10]

    How to do it: Wash your clothes in the warmest/hottest setting recommended for your clothing, and dry completely. Wash your dishes in the hottest water possible, but use a dishwasher if possible, because it can wash dishes and steam them. Water used in hand washing may not be hot enough to kill all bacteria. Use a floor, household, or handheld steamer to steam items such as curtains, mattresses, couches, and other surfaces where you can't spray disinfectants.

7. **Open windows**. Proper ventilation helps keep bacteria, viruses, and other pollutants out of indoor air. Research shows that ventilation and air flow can impact how diseases spread indoors. In more stagnant air, disease is more likely to spread. Effective ventilation can also reduce moisture. Bacteria and viruses are more likely to grow and spread in damp indoor spaces.[11]

    How to do it: Open windows as often as possible to bring in fresh air. If you're at work or in a public place, this is especially important. The CDC recommends opening windows at home, in the office, and when using public or shared transportation.

The Two-Step Cleaning Product Toss

Hopefully by now, you're convinced that most cleaning products are suspect until proven otherwise, and perhaps you've cleaned up a few stains on your carpet using baking soda and vinegar instead of harsh cleaners. But how do you deal with all the cleaning products you've accumulated over the years in your home? Do you need to throw out the laundry detergent first or the window cleaner?

First, I ask clients to think about which cleaning products they use most often. This tends to be things like hand soap, countertop cleaners, and laundry detergent—products that might get used multiple times per day. It's so easy to just start there and switch those right away. Replace both with a safer brand and *bam*—you've already made a big difference. Second, I ask clients about their health issues: Does someone in the home have allergies? Irritated skin? Respiratory issues? If there are health issues in the home, that is our next line of attack. Sometimes, once we replace the most used cleaners, clients will notice health improvements already. But if not, we start removing the harshest cleaners linked to some of these health problems right away. I suggest clients remove oven cleaner, tile cleaners, and their air fresheners if they haven't done that already.

At that point, I also check in with clients about how they are feeling about the DIY life. If clients have tried a few DIY products at this point, I then ask them: Are you finding it enjoyable? Or is it a pain in the rear? If it's painful, no need to continue! It's perfectly fine to use one of the safer brands, and you may even find that you end up saving money that way, which is surprising because many of the safer brands are more expensive. But many of them also come in concentrated solutions that can last quite a long time. I bought a safer laundry detergent that cost $30, which of course sounds like a lot! But since the solution was so concentrated, it lasted six months. Quite a feat for a family of five that does quite a bit of laundry!

Slightly greener cleaning assessment

When you've got the micro changes in Chapter 10 under your belt and gotten comfortable with a few of the simple DIY products from Chapter 11, it's time to take the next step. Together we will figure out which cleaning products you can keep until your supply runs out and which ones you should immediately give away or dispose of safely.

Go and collect the box of cleaning products and supplies I asked you to gather earlier. Now that you've got everything, separate your products into three groups:

Group #1: Barely used (75 percent or more full)

Group #2: Halfway through (about 50 percent full)

Group #3: Nearly gone (less than 30 percent full)

For Group #1: Give these away! (Or dispose of them safely—see Resources section.)

For Group #2: You can use these up if the product does not contain any of the following:

Glycol ethers (including 2-butoxyethanol and diethylene glycol)

Dyes

Fragrances (including synthetic musk)

Alkylphenol ethoxylates

Ethanolamines (DEA, MEA, TEA)

Quaternary ammonium compounds

Butyl cellusolve

Ammonia

Chlorinated phenol

Petroleum (including propane or isobutane or kerosene)

Bleach

* If you can't tell what ingredients are in your cleaners, you can try to go on the company's website to see if they list their ingredients there. If not, when in doubt, throw it out (responsibly, of course)!

If you do decide to still use them up, follow the steps in "Safely Using Your Emergency Stash" for how to safely use them.

For Group #3: You *can* use these up, but you could also consider adding these to your "emergency stash" or simply disposing of these products safely. (See box for details.)

SAFELY USING YOUR EMERGENCY STASH

I know that it's difficult to give a bunch of expensive products away, no matter how harmful they may be to your health. I keep bleach and carpet stain remover in my house for extra large or extremely dirty emergencies. If you'd like to use up what's left of the conventional cleaning products you have—or keep a couple of heavy hitters around for those really gross messes—here are a few tips for making these cleaners a little healthier for your family.

→ Dilute cleaning supplies (if instructions allow).

→ Use only what's needed to get the job done.

→ Clean with open windows (and doors if possible!).

→ Use gloves and/or goggles. This is especially important for cleaning products with chemicals that may harm or penetrate skin and eyes. Check warning labels for safety precautions.

→ Avoid antibacterial products. According to the American Medical Association, if your family is generally healthy, there is no need to use antibacterial products. In fact, using antibacterial ingredients, such as triclosan, can contribute to antibiotic-resistant "superbugs."

→ Keep children away from conventional cleaning products.

→ NEVER mix bleach with vinegar, ammonia, or other acids when cleaning. Combining these products can form deadly fumes. Check labels
to see if bleach or ammonia is used in the product. For instance, don't
use a bleach-containing toilet scrub with a window or multipurpose
cleaner that contains ammonia.

If you have any oven cleaners in your cupboards, toss them immediately. Oven cleaners are full of harmful ingredients, such as lye (caustic soda), ethylene glycol, and methylene chloride. These ingredients are linked to asthma and other respiratory problems and possibly cancer.

Out with the old (toxins) in with the new (houseplants)

Now that you've gotten rid of your most toxic cleaners, you might be ready to start bringing in some houseplants that are good for your health! A study from NASA found that some houseplants can remove up to 87 percent of indoor toxins within twenty-four hours.[1] Even if you've never had a green thumb, you might be motivated to do so now, huh? If you need any more convincing, studies have also shown that indoor plants can boost mood, concentration, and productivity and reduce stress.[2]

Here are a few houseplants from the NASA study, listed by their common and scientific names, along with their health benefits:

Spider plant (*Chlorophytum comosum*): Filters out carbon monoxide
    and formaldehyde.

Aloe vera (*Aloe barbadensis*): Filters formaldehyde and benzene.

English ivy (*Hedera helix*): Soaks up carcinogens from second-hand smoke.

Peace lily (*Spathiphyllum*): Has one of the highest transpiration rates; removes benzene, acetone, and trichloroethylene.

Golden pothos (*Epipremnum aureum*): One of the most effective at removing formaldehyde; also eliminates carbon monoxide.

Boston fern (*Nephrolepis exaltata*): Acts as a natural humidifier and eliminates formaldehyde.

Snake plant (*Sansevieria trifasciata*): Takes in carbon monoxide and releases oxygen during the night; filters formaldehyde.

Dracaena (*Dracaena deremensis*): Filters out trichloroethylene from solvents and varnishes.

Bamboo palm (*Chamaedorea seifrizii*): One of the best air filters for benzene and trichloroethylene and a great humidifier.

Dragon tree (*Dracaena marginata*): Known for its purifying properties; pulls xylene, benzene, toluene, and formaldehyde from the air but it is toxic to pets.

Whatever houseplants you decide to purchase, if you have pets, always make sure that you check to see if they are pet-friendly, as some plants that are just fine for humans are toxic to animals.

Moving forward

I hope by now you've implemented one or two (or perhaps several) tips from this part to reduce dust and improve air quality—well done! Take a

moment to appreciate the changes you've made. If you haven't yet implemented the full cleaning product cleanout, not to worry. You can always
come back to it later. The most important thing is that you stick with the
changes you've made, perhaps adding to them bit by bit as you go.

Seasonal cleaning

At this point, I also share a seasonal cleaning checklist with clients.
It's a great way to stay on track with keeping your home as dust- and
chemical-free as possible. If you miss one season (or even two!), no
worries. Just pick up where you left off and begin again. No judgment
and no pressure—just do what you can. Using the cleaning methods
and DIY recipes in Chapter 11, follow this seasonal cleaning checklist
to keep your house clean all year long. Bonus: Allergy and respiratory
symptoms may lessen by keeping a cleaner home and using products
that don't contain bleach or other respiratory irritants. You can also
use one of the safer brands recommended in the Resources section if
you are in a pinch and can't DIY it.

I also recommend following the Slightly Greener Method in each
category to clean and organize each season.

And an even bigger bonus? Your kids can help, and you don't have
to worry about them being exposed to harmful chemicals or fumes.
(They may not consider this a bonus!)

The first part of the chart contains the basics of seasonal cleaning. For an even deeper clean, you can also follow those listed in the
Deeper Clean section. As with all the tips in this book, remember,
it's about action, not perfection. Do what you can, and you can even

spread the tasks out over a longer period of time rather than trying to get them all done in a weekend. Check them off as you go—filling in a checkmark can be very satisfying and encourage you to do more! To print this checklist out, go to slightlygreenerbook.com.

Seasonal Cleaning Basics

SPRING	SUMMER	FALL	WINTER
Deep clean oven	Deep clean oven	Deep clean oven	Deep clean oven
Clean/organize pantry	Clean/organize pantry	Clean/organize pantry	Clean/organize pantry
Deep clean refrigerator	Deep clean refrigerator	Deep clean refrigerator	Deep clean refrigerator
Wash baseboards	Wash baseboards	Wash baseboards	Wash baseboards
Wash appliances	Wash appliances	Wash appliances	Wash appliances
Scrub tubs/ showers	Scrub tubs/ showers	Scrub tubs/ showers	Scrub tubs/ showers
Wash throw rugs	Wash throw rugs	Wash throw rugs	Wash throw rugs
Vacuum/damp mop all floors	Vacuum/damp mop all floors	Vacuum/damp mop all floors	Vacuum/damp mop all floors
Change furnace filter	Change furnace filter	Change furnace filter	Change furnace filter
*Vacuum and flip mattress	*Vacuum and flip mattress	*Vacuum and flip mattress	*Vacuum and flip mattress
Damp dust ceiling fans	Damp dust ceiling fans	Damp dust ceiling fans	Damp dust ceiling fans
Vacuum/wash vents	Vacuum/wash vents	Vacuum/wash vents	Vacuum/wash vents
Wipe down light switches	Wipe down light switches	Wipe down light switches	Wipe down light switches
Clean doorknobs	Clean doorknobs	Clean doorknobs	Clean doorknobs
Wash shower curtains	Wash shower curtains	Wash shower curtains	Wash shower curtains

SPRING	SUMMER	FALL	WINTER
Clean windows inside and outside	Vacuum lampshades	Clean windows inside and outside	Vacuum lampshades
Damp dust all surfaces	Damp dust all surfaces	Damp dust all surfaces	Damp dust all surfaces
Clean out freezer		Clean out freezer	

* If using a single-sided mattress, vacuum and rotate the mattress. If using a double-sided mattress, vacuum and have someone help you flip the mattress.

Deeper Clean

SPRING	SUMMER	FALL	WINTER
Spot clean walls	Spot clean walls	Spot clean walls	Spot clean walls
Touch-up paint	Touch-up paint	Touch-up paint	Touch-up paint
Clean cupboard shelves	Clean cupboard shelves	Clean cupboard shelves	Clean cupboard shelves
Clean under/ behind appliances	Wash window tracks	Clean under/ behind appliances	Wash window tracks

The following tips will help keep your house clean in-between those deep cleans:

Daily

Wipe off kitchen counters, table, and chairs

Wipe off stovetop

Vacuum kitchen floor

Vacuum playroom floor and areas where your family spends the most time

Twice per week (once a week at a minimum)

Vacuum bedrooms, family room, and children's play areas

Weekly

Clean microwave

Remove expired food/leftovers in refrigerator

Clean sponges

Damp mop kitchen floor

Vacuum and shake out floor mats

Dust and vacuum bedrooms and kids' play areas

Change bedsheets

Staying slightly greener

If you live in the United States or the United Kingdom, you might be familiar with the superstition of saying "rabbit, rabbit" first thing in the morning when you wake up on the first day of each month. It's meant to inspire good fortune for the remainder of the month, with the idea being that rabbits are good luck. This practice is believed to have originated in the early 1900s. President Franklin Delano Roosevelt said in 1935 that he was a devotee and uttered it every month. It's a useful practice, that monthly check-in.

But rather than doing a monthly check-in to ask for good luck, I'm more of a believer in *good choices*. The beginning of every month— heck, maybe even the beginning of every day—is a good opportunity to check in with yourself: *How am I doing? Have I veered off course?* Hopefully by now, *The Slightly Greener Method* has showed you that to be healthy people and wise consumers, we don't need to rely on luck. Instead, we have the power and the control to choose which foods and products we will buy and which ones we won't. (Hello, deal breakers.) But I bring this "rabbit, rabbit" tradition up because living a healthy lifestyle according to *The Slightly Greener Method* is a journey, and a regular practice of checking in is useful. There will be detours and pit stops. We might get lost and have to find our way back. There will be unexpected destinations.

As much as we might not like to admit it, we never really know what's around the next corner in life. But we are always in control of how we respond to any circumstance. You are in control of your environment, how you set up your home, and what products you use to do so. You're in charge of how you choose to feed your family. You get to decide which foods you will put on your plate and in your pantry. You have the power to avoid foods or products that fail to use safe ingredients. You get to decide what to slather on your skin (or what you will and won't put on your children). You get to decide which cleaning products to use and which ones to avoid.

And that matters. A lot actually.

But it *is* a journey, so don't give up if you veer off course. We all do. Whether it's a vacation (or a global pandemic), life happens, and sometimes our 80/20 dissolves and becomes more like 20/80. And that's OK.

Like Roosevelt did over eight decades ago, I like the idea of regular check-ins. Whether you say "rabbit, rabbit" monthly or do weekly or even quarterly check-ins, it's a good idea to revisit how you are doing on the Slightly Greener Method regularly. I've included the steps that I use on a weekly and quarterly basis in addition to my regular "why" check-in that you can use as inspiration for however you choose to regularly track your progress. Each month, ask yourself: What is my why? Is it the same as last month? Has it changed? As you twist and turn and meander down the journey that is your life, your why may change. That's fine! You may also find that your why stayed the same but you forgot to hold to your deal breakers. Or you caved when your kids begged for traditional microwave popcorn. That's OK too.

Use your regular check-ins—whatever they look like for you—as a time to reset and remember the bigger picture of your goals for optimal health. The specifics of the why, the deal breakers, and what the Slightly Greener Method lifestyle looks like as you bring it to fruition are entirely unique to you. And that's the beauty of this method: it's always here waiting for you to return to it, every time you forget or your why changes or you wake up and realize you ate an entire bag of Cheetos. It's all part of the process.

QUICK TIPS

→ Check the refrigerator and pantry weekly for expired items. I usually do this the night before garbage pickup.

→ When you toss something, replace it with a healthier item (check the Resources section for safer brands).

→ Keep a Sharpie in your bathroom to mark when you opened a product.

→ Keep a box of baking soda and a gallon of white vinegar under every bathroom sink in place of toilet bowl cleaner. (Remember: never combine them when storing them.) I always keep a bottle of my DIY window cleaner under each bathroom sink too.

→ Keep spray pumps from the cleaning products you dispose of or recycle. They come in handy when you DIY cleaning products.

→ Buy white vinegar in glass bottles whenever possible. For a quick vinegar spray for the DIY oven cleaner, carpet stain remover, or shower mold, you can just add distilled water when the bottle is half-empty. Just remove the plastic cap and attach the spray pump. You can also save the empty bottles for later DIY cleaners.

Quarterly cleanout

Makeup and personal care products

Check your shampoo, conditioner, other hair care products, shaving creams, lotions, and cosmetics. Also check old purses for old lipsticks and powders; you might be surprised how many you find! When in doubt, toss it out. I know it hurts, but better to be safe than sorry! And now that you're marking dates and checking items frequently, you'll feel great knowing what's safe to use and what's OK to toss.

Refrigerator and pantry items

Go through and do a more thorough search for expired items or items that may have been left half-opened and are no longer fresh or edible (Looking at you, my own kids!). This will give you lots of room to start replacing more foods and beverages with healthy choices!

Cleaning products

Isn't it surprising how fast we accumulate cleaning products? Some seem to appear in my cabinet that I have no recollection of buying. Go through this area quarterly, and either safely dispose of or recycle unwanted cleaning products, make a list of safer brands you need to buy, or DIY ones you want to make. It's amazing how good it feels to have organized cleaning cabinets so you can find exactly what you need.

Most important of all, when you toss something, replace it with a safer item

Do this as often as you can (check the Resources section for safer brands), and pretty soon you'll have a house that's the perfect shade of green for you!

When you fall off the wagon

Notice I said "when," not if. Because you *will* fall off the wagon. I still do, and I've learned that it's OK. Whether it's your own struggle to stay on course or a result of the people or circumstances around you, it's going to happen. We can't control everything 100 percent of the time, so there will be times when the store runs out of your favorite product, or you're traveling and can't find a safer shampoo, or my personal favorite—when my husband goes shopping and comes home with antibacterial soap!

When that happened, he said, "But look at the label. It says it's made with natural ingredients!"

Well, we can't win them all. He tries his best and does put in a lot of effort toward maintaining our slightly greener home, which is more than I can ask.

There may also be times when budget is an issue. My best advice for all these situations? Go back to the 80/20 rule: **If you can buy safer products 80 percent of the time, you don't have to worry about the other 20 percent of the time when you can't control the situation.** This way, you can still enjoy the occasional treat. Remember, this lifestyle isn't about complete deprivation or about making every change all at once. It's not all or nothing—it's about balance and what's right for your family. Can't do 80/20? Fine. It's totally OK to start with 60/40 and work your way up from there. What it *is* about is making small changes to start, which will eventually add up to a big change in detoxifying your home.

When you do get off track, just start right back up with the next small change. I think so many of us feel like we *have* to be perfect or that once we mess up, we've ruined it, so why bother? But deep down inside, we know that's not the way change works. All it takes is making the best *next* decision.

When your family isn't on board

My family has been living this lifestyle for over fifteen years now. When you hear me say that, you probably think that I've got this thing totally under control. That my family blissfully follows along with whatever I buy.

False.

Just a few months ago, my teenage girls asked me, "When can we have a normal home and just buy regular stuff?" This happens every once in a while, and while I may or may not have lost my cool over the antibacterial soap and dishwashing detergent my husband brought home, I reminded my girls that we buy *mostly* safer stuff. And in the grand scheme of things, choices about hand and dish soap don't personally affect them too much.

I've learned some pretty good strategies for those situations when my family isn't on board. When I first started, I know I went too far and drove myself *and* my family crazy. And it was clear that was the totally wrong approach. Once I began to realize that I had to replace things *slowly* to get my family used to it, it got much easier. (And in some cases, I didn't even tell them unless it affected them directly!) For example, my older daughter loves Pop-Tarts, so rather than saying "no more Pop-Tarts ever again," I bought a safer brand for her that contains natural colorings such as beet root powder, rather than artificial colors like FD&C Red No. 40. I also replaced things such as Froot Loops with a safer brand that uses natural colorings too.

Don't quit. It gets easier, I promise

To be honest, I am a candle-loving, Milk Dud–eating, noncooking kind of gal. So that's why throughout this book, I have said, *If I can live this lifestyle, so can you.* I am truly just a mom who has figured it out, and I will help you do it too. You'll be surprised how automatic it will become to know which products you can buy and which ones to avoid and how quickly you'll be able to read labels at the store. When you follow the steps below, it will be easy to know where to start when it comes to detoxing your home, and just take it from there.

▸ **Remember your why.** When you keep this in mind, the decisions will be easy.

▸ **Start by deciding what your deal-breaker ingredients.** When you see that ingredient(s) on the label, avoid it. That will save a lot of time when shopping!

▸ **Once you feel comfortable avoiding your deal-breaker ingredients, move on to ingredients of concerns you'd like to avoid.**

This has been a journey for my family too. My kids are older now, and they are making their own choices. My son Eric's attention issues were our wake-up call and the catalyst that set us on this path. I was able to help him tremendously by changing some key components of his environment. Now he's twenty-three, and I'm not making many choices for him. He's not perfect; he's away at college and loves to eat junk food and drink beer, like just about every college kid! He doesn't always make the best decisions, but for the most part, he listens to me and takes my messages to heart.

In fact, Eric seems to be the one in my home who listens the most closely to what I say. (Well, when it comes to this at least.) Not only did he see and feel the results back in second grade, but he still sees an impact today. When he gets sick, he knows what supplements to take and uses natural remedies to feel better, because he knows what helps him heal faster and how to support his body while he recovers. Now that he's living away from home, he still tries to incorporate a slightly greener lifestyle as often as he can. I recently asked him what he does at school to have a less-toxic apartment, and I loved his answer. He said while it is challenging to buy safer products and foods on a regular basis while he's away, he has realized it's more about the things he *doesn't* do than what he *does* do. For example, he doesn't use plastic cooking utensils or food storage containers in the kitchen. He also doesn't use candles or air fresheners, which he used in the past. And as far as ingredients, he knows that his deal-breaker ingredient for shampoo is sodium lauryl sulfate, so he buys a sulfate-free shampoo. And I love that he keeps vinegar and baking soda under his bathroom sink to use as a toilet bowl cleaner and uses the DIY window cleaner for his mirror. Even though I'm not there in his college apartment telling him what to do and what to buy—or not buy—he's made some really healthy choices on his own! And he's on a journey too. The choices he makes at thirty-three and forty-three and beyond will probably look much different from the ones he's making now at twenty-three.

And that's great. As his mom, I'm incredibly proud.

AFTER THE SLIGHTLY GREENER METHOD

Use this book as a reference as you move toward your perfect shade of green. Once you feel confident in your initial changes, go back through the book as your why changes or as you meet your goals and are ready to move on to add more changes. This is your unique journey, and the fun part is moving on to the next level!

The Slightly Greener Method isn't over once you finish this book or complete the cleanouts. You will have the most success with this lifestyle if you view it as a constant evolution.

As I shared in the opening page of this book, if there was one quote that distilled the essence of this method, it would be one of my favorites from Maya Angelou:

"Do the best you can until you know better. Then when you know better, do better."

I hope that in these pages, you've found research, tips, and tools that have instructed you in a way that makes you feel empowered, like you know better.

Now, the way forward on this path is up to you. Perhaps the most challenging part will be remembering that the goal isn't "the best" or "finished" or "first place in the Slightly Greener Method" or anything even close to that. The goal is simple: do better, whatever that looks like for you.

For me, and I hope for you too, better is a fun place to be.

Life is for living. And to me, that means tossing parabens, yes. But it also means tossing back the occasional Twinkie. And loving every bite.

Acknowledgments

The phrase "it takes a village" can work with so many things, including writing a book. And I am so grateful for so many people who have been a part of mine as I sit down to write these acknowledgments.

There are not enough words to thank my family. For my husband, James, thank you for your unwavering support and for encouraging me to do the hard things I never thought I could do. And for putting up with a messy house and having to fend for yourself and the kids for dinner many a night. You supported and trusted me through many crazy twists and turns through my business to get to this point of my dream of writing a book, and I couldn't be more grateful.

To my children, Eric, Kaylee, and Lyndsey: this journey began because of you, and you each deserve so much credit and respect for sharing your stories in this book. You have supported me more than you'll ever know, with your patience and understanding, your words of encouragement, and your excitement for this work as well as the ventures we have taken on as a family. You have grown into amazing young adults, and you have taught me more than you'll ever know.

And to my parents, I'm struggling to find the right words, because "thank you" doesn't seem to be enough. Your belief in me allowed me to believe that I can be and do anything. You have always led by example and taught me the importance of kindness, generosity, perseverance, and hard work in all that I do.

To my agent, Lucinda Halpern, you saw my vision for this book and crafted it even better and stronger. I'm forever grateful for your insight, support, and encouragement, and for taking a chance on me.

Endless gratitude to my editor, Anna Michels, at Sourcebooks. Thank you so much for believing in me and in my vision for this book. Your invaluable feedback and input helped make this book even better than I could have imagined. I'm so grateful for you and the entire Sourcebooks team for bringing this book to life.

Heartfelt thanks to Jackie Ashton. I'm so grateful for your support, collaboration, editing, and so much more. Thank you for helping me get the words out of my head and onto paper.

To Meghan Stevenson, thank you for creating an amazing book proposal, and for getting my voice and vision clear.

A huge heartfelt thank you to Super Connector Media: Chris Winfield (this all started when you told me that I have a responsibility to get my message out!), Jen Gottleib, Angela Bonnici, Olivia Moore, and Catherine Boardman. Your support, advice, and encouragement have meant to the world to me, and I'm so grateful for the opportunities you've given me to share my message. And Ashley Bernardi, I'm so grateful to have you on my team, and for helping me launch this book out into the world.

I have been blessed in having supportive mentors along the way, also: Todd Herman, Kathy Gulinello, Tricia Brouk, Kate Santichen, Paula Rizzo, and Farnoosh Torabi. Thank you so much for your guidance!

Working with so many amazing people has had a bigger impact on me than they will ever know.

And last but definitely not least, my clients and Slightly Greener family: thank you for letting me share your stories. Your kind words and support along the way have kept me motivated and made my purpose even stronger. This book is possible because of you.

Appendix A

Resources

Safer shopping for baby

Toys

- ▸ Avoid hand-me-downs where it's difficult to know what ingredients were used to make the product.
- ▸ Avoid any toys made with PVC/vinyl or BPA.
- ▸ Avoid toys made using formaldehyde glues and toxic finishes.
- ▸ Look for safer options: food-grade silicone, untreated natural hardwood, or 100 percent natural rubber.

Teethers

- ▸ Updated regulations have now banned five types of phthalates.
- ▸ Some teethers and soft baby/toddler toys can still contain undesirable chemicals such as PVC/vinyl or BPA, so avoid those!
- ▸ Look for safer options: food-grade silicone, untreated natural hardwood, or 100 percent natural rubber.

Baby clothes and crib sheets

▸ Avoid hand-me-downs, as clothes could have been treated with harsh chemicals (detergents and stain removers, for example) or could have harmful elements in them that aren't obvious to you.

▸ Baby clothes (and all clothes) can contain flame retardants, toxic residues from pesticides, formaldehyde, and plastic. Instead, look for clothes, sheets, and towels that are made with natural fibers: bamboo, hemp, and cotton.

Baby oil, baby powder, and petroleum jelly

▸ The reality is babies really don't need these products. If they have dry skin and need moisturizing beyond everyday nontoxic lotion, coconut oil is a great (and safe) option. I also recommend parents use a safer brand of diaper cream instead of petroleum jelly.

▸ As we learned, mineral oil is harmful to children, and the talc often found in baby powder has been linked to ovarian cancer. Baby powder has also been recalled over fears that it contained cancer-causing asbestos.[1]

Baby shampoos, lotions, sunscreens, and laundry detergent

▸ Be careful with these products. I only suggest purchasing the safer brands listed later in this section. Many "pediatrician recommended" products marketed for babies include some harmful ingredients that I recommend avoiding.

▸ Babies don't really need sunscreen. Most contain ingredients they shouldn't be exposed to, and their skin is thinner, making the ingredients easier to absorb. Instead, I suggest using hats and long-sleeved clothing or moving them inside or into the shade when it's too sunny.

Furniture (like bouncy seats, swings, playpens), car seats, and baby carriers

▸ Stay away from any product that contains polyurethane foam or PVC/vinyl.

▸ Make sure the plastic is BPA-free.

▸ Buy a crib mattress that is made with natural materials like 100 percent latex, wool, or organic cotton.

Ingredients to avoid based on health issues

ADHD

MSG	Fragrance
BPA	Artificial colors
BHA/BHT	Natural and artificial flavors
HFCS	Methylisothiazolinone

Weight

MSG	Carrageenan
BPA	Artificial sweeteners

Parabens   Fragrance

Phthalates

Hormones/endocrine disruptors

BHA/BHT   Phthalates

Fragrance   Parabens

BPA

Cancer

Artificial colors   SLS

Artificial sweeteners   Fragrance

BHA/BHT   1,4-dioxane

HFCS   Formaldehyde releasers

Carrageenan   Parabens

Brain health

MSG   Methylisothiazolinone

BPA   Fragrance

Artificial sweeteners

Eczema and allergies

SLS   Phthalates

Fragrance   Methylisothiazolinone

Pregnancy

Artificial sweeteners   MSG

Fragrance   Parabens

Phthalates

* *Keep in mind this is not a complete list; only ingredients discussed in this book are listed here. Diet and lifestyle changes also play an important role. Talk to your healthcare professional if any of these conditions are of concern, and don't go off any medication unless under a doctor's supervision.*

Safer brands

How to use this guide

It's hard to know which products are truly safer unless you've spent hundreds of hours learning about ingredients, hidden toxins, and the meaning behind terms on labels. The good news is I've been studying this for over ten years, and I have found lots of amazing brands and products!

This guide was created from research I have compiled over the last several years, with brands I have personally used with my own family or those for which I have carefully vetted the ingredients.

How do products meet my criteria?

- No MLM or direct sales products are allowed; I do not endorse or promote any direct sales products.
- The product has clearly labeled ingredients or ones that I've been able to get from the manufacturer.

- No products have toxins from my "ingredients to avoid" lists.
- I have carefully vetted the ingredients of or personally used and love the product.

Tips for using this guide

- This guide is divided into several categories and subcategories for ease of use. For example, the food section has subcategories such as organic dairy, safer candy, etc.
- Website links change frequently, so it is possible that some may no longer work. Please email my team at support@slightlygreener .com, and we will work on getting it fixed right away.

Where to find these products

- Visit the company website and see if they have a "Find a Store" or "Find a Retailer" tab in their menu (stores change merchandise and links quickly, so be sure to check company websites often).
- Search the product name you're looking for on Amazon. Many of these products are available there.
- Check sites that may carry these products at a better price, such as Thrive Market or Vitacost.

Organic dairy/yogurt

Stonyfield: Organic yogurt, milk and cream, and frozen treats

Horizon Organic: Organic dairy

Organic Valley: Organic dairy

Wallaby Organic: Organic yogurt, Greek yogurt, and sour cream

Maple Hill Creamery: 100 percent grass-fed and organic yogurt, Greek
    yogurt, drinkable yogurt, and kefir

Organic candy

YumEarth: Naturally flavored (from fruits and vegetables) candy;
    certified organic, 100 percent vegan, GMO-free, allergen-free,
    gluten-free. Also wheat, casein, and dairy-free. These candies
    are delicious!

Theo Chocolate: Organic/Non-GMO Project verified chocolate and
    candies, family owned

Surf Sweets: Organic gummies and jelly beans free of artificial dyes,
    Non-GMO Project verified, allergy friendly

Wholesome: Organic DelishFish (organic, gluten-free, no artificial
    colors or flavors, non-GMO, vegan gummy fish)

Gnosis Chocolate: Organic, gluten-free, soy-free, dairy-free, non-
    GMO, and ethically sourced chocolate (raw cacao)

Cookies

Thrive Tribe Paleo Cookies: Whether you follow a paleo diet or not,
    these cookies taste great and use whole-food ingredients

Back to Nature: Non-GMO Project verified cookies

Organic snacks and cereals

Driscoll's: Organic (and conventionally grown) berries

NOW Foods: Health foods and snacks

EnviroKidz: Cereals and snack bars; USDA Certified Organic,

Non-GMO Project verified, vegetarian, and certified gluten-free; find discounted at Costco, Walmart, BJ's, Sam's Club, Big Lots, and other club or warehouse stores

Nature's Path: Certified organic cereals, granola, toaster pastries, baking mixes, hot cereals, and snack bars

Cascadian Farm: Organic, non-GMO cereals, granola bars, fruit spreads, and more

Cedar's Foods: Hummus, salsa, dips, pita chips, salads, and more. Their all-natural hummus is Non-GMO Project verified.

Enjoy Life Foods: Snacks and baking mixes that are free from the top eight allergens, including gluten, peanuts, and soy; non-GMO

Newman's Own Organics: Organic products including pretzel snacks, cookies, dried fruit, coffee, tea, oils, vinegars and salad dressings, and pet food. Ingredients used in all their products are grown on farms that have not used artificial fertilizers or pesticides for three years or more.

SimpleMills: Gluten-free, soy-free, gum-free, paleo-friendly, non-GMO

Elemental Superfood: Crumbles and seedbars that are free of gluten and dairy and are full of good fats and high-quality protein

Mary's Gone Crackers: Organic, gluten-free, non-GMO crackers, cookies, and snacks

Arrowhead Mills: Organic baking mixes, cereals, flours, and nut butters; many products Non-GMO Project verified (many more of their products are enrolled); gluten-free options

Thrive Tribe: Paleo-friendly and gluten-, dairy-, and grain-free, non-GMO bars, bites, and coconut chips

Grains and breads

Bob's Red Mill: Grains, beans, seeds, mixes, granola, flours and
meals, and gluten-free items. Most (not all) are organic and non-
GMO; be sure to check the label

Lundberg Family Farms: White rice (lowest level of arsenic), grains,
snacks, baking products

Rudi's Organic Bakery: 100 percent organic, GMO-free bread, rolls,
and other baked goods

Eden Foods: Whole grains, cereals, condiments, oil and vinegar,
pasta, snack foods; BPA-free packaging; BPA-free cans for low-
acid foods; glass jars for tomato products; caps with protective
sealants

Back to the Roots: Organic cereals

Baking

SimpleMills: Non-GMO Project verified baking mixes

Wholesome: Organic and natural sugars (cane, powdered, brown,
sucanat, coconut, turbinado) and frosting; Non-GMO Project
verified, gluten-free, no HFCS or artificial colors or flavors

Arrowhead Mills: Organic baking mixes, cereals, flours, and nut
butters; many products Non-GMO Project verified; gluten-free
options

Rumford: Non-GMO Project verified and aluminum-free baking
powder and cornstarch

Clabber Girl: Non-GMO Project verified and aluminum-free baking
soda

Organic soups/broths/stocks

Imagine: Soups, stocks, and gravies that are free from harmful pesticides, preservatives, and GMO ingredients

Pacific Foods: Organic broths, stocks, soups, and sauces

Amy's: A large variety of foods that are organic and GMO-free;
canned soups are BPA-free

Note: Be sure to buy foods that don't need to be microwaved as much
as possible, but if you can't, remove from the plastic and put in a
microwave-safe dish first.

Nut butters

KALOT Superfood: Almond, cashew, and sunflower butters, using
only real fruit, nuts or seeds, and spice for different flavors

Justin's: Almond, cashew, and peanut butters made with organic
ingredients

Organic coconut oil

Nutiva: Organic and Non-GMO Project verified coconut, hemp, and
chia products; some certified gluten-free

Organic juices

Apple & Eve: Certified organic juices; juices not in their organic line
come from produce grown without pesticides

Leaf & Love: Zero-sugar juice boxes, Non-GMO Project verified, no
artificial ingredients

Pizza crust

Cali'flour Foods: Gluten-free, low-carb pizza crusts made from
    cauliflower, available in several flavors including jalapeño, sweet
    red pepper, and original Italian. They are also amazing when cut
    and used with dips or soups!

Hummus and guacamole

Lilly's: Non-GMO certified hummus

Hope Foods: Organic, non-GMO certified hummus, guacamole, and
    vegan dips

Roots: Non-GMO certified hummus

Cedar's Foods: Non-GMO certified hummus

Trader Joe's Organic Hummus

Wholly Guacamole: Premade guacamole with few ingredients

Organic baby/toddler/kids foods

Happy Family Organics

Sprout Organic Foods

Serenity Kids

Tuna

Safe Catch: lowest mercury of any brand; non-GMO, BPA-free

Chips and crackers

Frontera: Non-GMO Project verified tortilla chips and other
    Mexican foods

Luke's Organic: Organic, gluten-free, Non-GMO Project verified,
    vegan potato and multigrain chips

Kettle Brand: Most potato chip flavors are Non-GMO Project veri-
    fied (check bags for info)

Food Should Taste Good: Non-GMO Project verified multigrain
    tortilla chips and brown rice crackers

Garden of Eatin': All-natural chips, many of which are organic and/
    or Non-GMO Project verified

Back to Nature: Cereal, cookies, and crackers with many organic
    and/or Non-GMO Project verified

Jackson's Honest: Organic and non-GMO tortilla chips and potato chips

Natural sweeteners

SweetLeaf: Stevia sweeteners in powdered, liquid, and syrup form

NOW Foods: Organic stevia sweetener in powder, liquid, and packets

Pure Via: Stevia liquid sweetener

Sweet Dreams: Brown rice syrup

Nature Botanicals: 100% pure yacon syrup

Popcorn

Ready to eat

Angie's Boom Chicka Pop

Sage Valley

Trader Joe's

O Organics

Kernels

Arrowhead Mills

Eden Foods

Great Northern

NOW Foods

Trader Joe's

Organic ice cream

Luna & Larry's Coconut Bliss: Organic, dairy-free, gluten-free, soy-free, and Non-GMO Project verified

Stoneyfield: Organic frozen yogurt and frozen yogurt bars

Whole Foods 365 Brand Organic Ice Cream

Organic wines

EcoVine Wine Club: Membership club that offers organic, sulfite-free, vegan, and biodynamic wines (can be canceled anytime with no penalty)

Dry Farm Wines: Membership club that offers organic wines, low sulfite, low sugar, mycotoxin- and mold-free, paleo, low/slow carb, sugar-free, carb-free, and ketogenic-friendly (can be cancelled anytime with no penalty)

Sauces

San-J: Non-GMO Project verified tamari soy sauces

Lunch meat, hot dogs, bacon, etc.

Applegate Farms

FOOD-BUYING TIPS

→ The Non-GMO Shopping Guide is another great resource for finding organic, non-GMO foods.

→ Don't forget to check out manufacturer websites for coupons!

→ Many of these brands are also available at Thrive Market for a deep discount of sometimes up to 50 percent off.

→ Also check discount sites like Vitacost.

Cookware and food storage

Cookware

Always Pan: A nonstick pan that uses ceramic coating (includes spatula and steamer basket)

All-Clad: Stainless steel cookware (D3 stainless collection)

Xtrema Cookware: Nonstick cookware with ceramic coating. They include results from over fifty product testing reports over twelve years that show the products are free of extractable lead, cadmium, and other heavy metals under the U.S. government guidelines for heavy metals and chemicals.

Lodge: Cast iron cookware

Cooking utensils

Midori Way: Organic bamboo cutting board; eco-friendly and free of
formaldehyde and toxic dyes

Neet: Organic bamboo cooking and serving utensils; eco-friendly
utensils made of bamboo with vegetable oil coating

Food storage

Pyrex: Glass food storage containers with plastic lids

Bayco: Glass food storage containers with leak-proof snap lids

Wean Green: Glass food storage for food prep, snacks, lunch tubs, and
more; polypropylene #5 plastic lids with food-grade silicone seals

Lifefactory: Glass food storage with protective silicone sleeves

Rubbermaid: Glass containers with EasyFindLids

*Note: When using glassware with plastic lids, cool food off before placing
the plastic lid on, and don't let food touch the lid.*

Mixing bowls

Finedine: Heavy-duty stainless steel nesting mixing bowls for mixing
and food storage with airtight lids

Avacraft: Heavy-duty stainless steel mixing bowls with lids, handles,
and measurement lines; lids come in different colors

Personal Care Products and Cosmetics

Cosmetics

All Natural Cosmetics   Nvey Eco

100% Pure   W3ll People

Annmarie Skin Care   Juice Beauty

RMS Beauty   Real Purity

Skin care

Face

Beauty by Earth   Nourish Organic

Green Envee   By Valenti Organics

100% Pure   Real Purity

Alitura Naturals   Cocoon Apothecary

Organic to Green   Gressa

Ursa Major   Soapwalla

Suki   Juice Beauty

Carina Organics   French Girl Organics

Abbey Brown   Annmarie

Body

100% Pure   By Valenti Organics

Green Envee   Real Purity

Alitura Naturals   Cocoon Apothecary

Aubrey Organics   Juice Beauty

Organic to Green   French Girl Organics

Ursa Major

Juice Beauty

Nourish Organic

Personal Care Products (Children and Baby)

Dolphin Organics

100% Pure

Aubrey Organics

Earth Mama Organics

Green Envee

California Baby

Bath and Shower

100% Pure

Vermont Soap

Ursa Major

Aubrey Organics

Carina Organics

Abbey Brown

Nourish Organic

MamaSuds

Cocoon Apothecary

Hair Care

Beauty by Earth

100% Pure

Aubrey Organics

Real Purity

Juice Organics

ren jord

Toothpaste

Dr. Bronner's

Primal Life Organics

Pretty Frank

Redmond's Earthpaste and
    Earthpowder

Soaps

Vermont Soap

Dr. Bronner's

By Valenti Organics

Redmond's Earthcure

Hand soap

Carina Organics   Vermont Soap

By Valenti Organics

Scents

Aftelier Perfumes   Pour le Monde

Kate's Magik   French Girl Organics

Natural Perfumer's Guild   By Valenti Organics

Nail polish

Piggy Paint   Acquarella

Honeybee Gardens   Suncoat

SOPHi   Butter London

Deodorant

Pretty Frank   Soapwalla

Primal Life Organics   Ursa Major

Lip balm

Pretty Frank   Soapwalla

Eco Lips   Juice Beauty

Dr. Bronner's   Annmarie

Green Envee

Ellovi

Beauty by Earth

Abbey Brown

Lip scrub

By Valenti Organics   Henné Organics

French Girl Organics

Self-tanner

Beauty by Earth

Shaving cream

Aubrey Organics   Ursa Major

Gluten-free

Afterglow Cosmetics   Annmarie

Aubrey Organics

Sunscreen and insect repellent

Sunscreen

Badger   Kiss My Face

Beauty by Earth   All Good

Goddess Garden Organics   Tropical Sands

SPF lip protection

Eco Lips   Tropical Sands

Badger   All Good

After-sun care

Beauty by Earth   Badger

Insect repellent

Skedattle   Fit Organic

Mighty No Bitey   Flick the Tick

Hand sanitizers

CleanWell: sanitizing sprays,   Spinster Sisters Co.
    foams, and travel wipes   Pranarom

Dr. Bronner's   Saavy Naturals

Elyptol: hand sanitizing gel,
    spray, and wipes

Cleaning products

Laundry

Tandi's Naturals   Fit Organic: Laundry detergent

Molly's Suds   and stain remover

MamaSuds: Wool dryer ball in   Eco-Me
    place of fabric softener

Dishwasher detergent/dish soap

Nature Clean   Vermont Soap   Better Life: Dish

Earth Friendly   MamaSuds   soap and dish-
    Products   Fit Organic   washer gel

Furniture polish/dusting spray

Truce: Wood cleaner   Eco-Me: Wood polish

Toilet bowl cleaner

MamaSuds   Greenshield Organic

Air freshening

Arm & Hammer: Baking soda   Himalayan salt lamp

Aussan Natural   Vermont Soap

Mold and mildew

Attitude   Eco-Me

Concrobium

Stainless steel cleaner

Eco-Me

Floor cleaners

Fit Organic

Truce: Wood cleaner for furniture and wood/laminate floors

Eco-Me: Wood polish for furniture and wood/laminate floors; floor
    cleaner

Aunt Fannie's

All-purpose cleaners

Vermont Soap: Liquid Sunshine spray and castile liquid soaps

MamaSuds: All-purpose cleaner and castile soap

Fit Organic

Poppy's

Greenshield Organic

Dr. Bronner's

Eco-Me

Aunt Fannie's: All-purpose cleaning vinegar and wipes

Glass cleaners

Greenshield Organic   Aunt Fannie's

Calcium, lime, and rust remover

Fit Organic

Nonchlorine bleach

Ecover   Molly's Suds

Seventh Generation

Candles

Bluecorn Beeswax   Pure Plant Home (coconut wax)

Honey Candles

Beeswax Candle Works

Bee Hive Candles

Big Dipper Wax Works

For DIY cleaners

Essential oils

Mountain Rose Herbs   Green Envee

Essential oil diffusers

PureSpa   GreenAir

Riverock

Himalayan salt lamp

Himalayan Salt Shop

Glass spray bottles

Amazon: Amber or cobalt glass bottles (or reuse empty glass vinegar
    bottles)

Castile soap

Dr. Bronner's   Vermont Soap Organics

Furniture and mattresses

Mattresses

Happsy

Avocado

Naturepedic

Birch

Furniture without flame retardants

If you're buying new furniture and would like to avoid flame-retardant chemicals, these are brands that have phased them out:

La-Z-Boy	Futon Shop
Ashley Furniture	Scandinavian Designs
Room & Board	Dania Furniture
Crate & Barrel	Endicott Home Furnishings
IKEA	Eco-Terric
Ethan Allen	Furnature
West Elm	Green Sofas
Pottery Barn, Pottery Barn Kids	EcoBalanza
Design Within Reach	Naturepedic

Infant and child products that do not contain flame-retardant chemicals

Naturepedic: Changing pads, baby and kids' mattresses

Combi USA: Strollers, car seats (see their statement on car seats on the bottom of their FAQ page)

MamaDoo Kids: Playpens, mattress toppers

BabyBjörn: Baby carriers and jumpers

Britax: Strollers, car seats, accessories

Carter's: Infant and children's clothing

Inglesina: High chairs and strollers

Kolcraft: Bassinets, walkers, strollers, nursery furniture

Peg Perego: Strollers, high chairs, booster chairs, bike seats, accessories

Websites to help you shop safer

Environmental Working Group

Dirty Dozen Produce List

Clean 15 Produce List

Tap Water Database

Water Filter Guide

Find local CSAs and farmers markets

LocalHarvest: Find local CSAs and farmers markets

GreenPeople: Guide to local CSAs

Eat Well Guide: A directory of sustainably raised meat, poultry,
    eggs, and dairy

Farmers Market Coalition: farmersmarketcoalition.org

Local Harvest: localharvest.org/search

Local Farm Markets: www.localfarmmarkets.org

National Farmer's Market Directory: ams.usda.gov/local-food
    -directories/farmers markets

Find local, sustainably raised food

Eatwild (eatwild.com): Online directory of local grass-fed meat and
    dairy

Heritage Foods (heritagefoods.com)

Seasonal Food Guide: Makes buying in-season easy. Find out what
    produce is available in your state throughout the year

Find healthier seafood

Mercury Calculator: See how much mercury is in the seafood you
    are consuming

Smart Seafood Buying Guide: The NRDC's five tips to buying safer
    seafood

Seafood Watch: How to find safer seafood that's been fished or farmed
    with less impact on the environment

Find food co-ops

Co-op Directory Service: coopdirectory.org/directory.htm

Cooperative Grocer Network: cooperativegrocer.coop

Local Harvest: localharvest.org/food-coops

Find natural foods and products at a discount

Thrive Market: Online membership store that carries natural and
    organic products at wholesale prices (be sure to check food and
    product labels carefully). Use this link to get your membership
    free for sixty days, plus twenty-five dollars off your first order.

Vitacost: Supplements and health care items at a discount; dedicated
    non-GMO brands have their own section here.

Find safer cosmetics and personal care products

Campaign for Safer Cosmetics: Find out if your favorite cosmetics
    companies have signed the pact for safer cosmetics

Cosmetics Database: The EWG's safety scoring of beauty products

All Natural Cosmetics (allnaturalcosmetics.com)

Vitacost (vitacost.com): Supplements, health items, non-GMO snacks

Thrive Market: Healthier products at wholesale prices

Sephora: Safer products are on their "Clean at Sephora" list

> *Note: Although they do have some safer products on this page, be sure to read the labels carefully and use your shopping cheat sheet to look for toxic ingredients in some of the brands they have listed.*

Find safer scents and perfume

Aftelier (afterlier.com)

Treehugger: Guide to natural perfumes

Apps

Food

Fooducate (Free): This app allows you to scan the barcodes on product labels to get nutrition info as well as letter grade food scores. It also has options that will help you meet your nutritional needs, including a FoodPoints value number to help you stay on track without counting calories. Available on iTunes and Google Play.

Find Me Gluten-Free (Free): Read reviews and find local restaurants, cafés, and grocery stores that serve gluten-free menu items. View menus, get directions, or even call straight from the app. Also includes a Products Beta! scanner to scan food labels to see if they contain gluten. Available on iTunes and Google Play.

Non-GMO Shopping Guide (Free): The Non-GMO Project is the only third-party non-GMO verification program in North America, and this app helps you know which brands to choose and which to avoid. Available on iTunes and Google Play.

Seafood Watch (Free): This app from the Monterey Bay aquarium helps you find sustainable options for seafood and sushi based on GPS location. You can also find the best choices in seafood that are also lower in contaminants and those that are high in omega-3 fatty acids. Available on iTunes and Google Play.

ShopWell (Free): Scan barcodes and see if the food is a good match for you. You can use it for conditions such as diabetes, high blood pressure, and celiac disease. You can also use it to avoid allergens or certain ingredients. Available on iTunes and Google Play.

Seasonal Food Guide (Free): Never wonder again if a food is in season in your area. This app lists over 140 fruits, veggies, legumes, nuts, and herbs to help you find seasonal, local food in your state. Available on iTunes and Google Play.

Harvest ($1.99): Ever wonder how to choose the best produce at the supermarket? This app will help! Harvest will tell you the best way to store your food and even incorporates the EWG's pesticide information. Available for iPhone only.

Food Additives 2 ($0.99): Search over 450 food additives to find out which ones are safer than others. The database doesn't require internet connection. Available for iPhone only.

Daily Blends: The Ultimate Green Smoothie App ($2.99): Over one hundred green smoothie recipes. Select your favorites, add them to a shopping list, and search for recipes you can customize and make with food you already have. Available on iTunes and Google Play.

Cosmetics

Think Dirty (Free): From the Campaign for Safe Cosmetics, simply scan a product's bar code to get safety info on the product as well as safer options. Available on iTunes and Google Play.

Nontoxic living

Detox Me (Free): Evaluate key areas of your daily life in six categories. This app helps you to detox and find safer products where you live and work. You can also track your progress to see how far you've come. The app contains over 270 tips to help you have a healthier home. Available on iTunes and Google Play.

Appendix B

Cheat Sheets

Use the cheat sheets below for quick and easy label checking while shopping. Visit the book website to print these out or download them to your phone.

Ingredients to Avoid in Food

INGREDIENT	FOUND IN	HEALTH EFFECTS
Natural flavors	Coffee creamer, oatmeal, fruit snacks, cereals, spices, beverages, soups, dairy products	• May hide ingredients such as MSG and gluten • Considered to be a proprietary formula so individual ingredients are not required to be listed
Artificial flavors	Candy, chips, crackers, salad dressings, ice cream, cereal, fruit juices, flavored yogurt, toothpaste, and medicines	• Considered to be a proprietary formula so individual ingredients are not required to be listed • Made up of chemicals that can include preservatives, solvents, and other additives

INGREDIENT	FOUND IN	HEALTH EFFECTS
High fructose corn syrup	Many processed foods, such as crackers, cookies, condiments, cereals, chips, jelly, and some vitamins	· Linked to diabetes, obesity, and metabolic disorder · Also linked to cancer and accelerated aging · GMO and possible mercury contamination
Monosodium glutamate	Most processed foods, such as chips, salad dressings, canned soups, sauces, flavored crackers, and in spices and flavorings (such as some taco seasonings and Accent flavor enhancer)	· Hides in over forty different ingredients · May excite neurons (nerve cells) to the point of cell death · May affect the development of the nervous system
Carrageenan	Dairy products such as ice cream, heavy whipping cream, ice cream, cottage cheese, and yogurt	· Linked to colitis and colon cancer · May contribute to weight gain · Interferes with beneficial flora in GI tract
Artificial sweeteners	Sugar-free and diet foods and beverages, such as diet soda, sugar-free jelly, sugar-free Jell-O, flavored water, and Pedialyte. Includes brand names Splenda, Sweet'N Low, Equal	· Linked to birth defects · May alter gut flora · Linked to neurological disorders, such as Alzheimer's and multiple sclerosis
BHA and BHT	Snack foods, cereal, processed meats, gum, beer, lining of food packages (will usually see "BHT added for freshness" on label)	· May be cancer causing · Sleep and behavior issues · Interferes with hormone function and may mimic estrogen
Benzoates	Foods and beverages such as soda, fruit juice, pickles, soy sauce, tomato sauce, and even in flavored water	· Linked to hyperactivity in children · Can form benzene (a known cancer causer) when combined with vitamin C

INGREDIENT	FOUND IN	HEALTH EFFECTS
Artificial colors	Cereals, medicines, candy, toothpaste, Popsicles, frosting, canned vegetables, ice cream	· Linked to hyperactivity · Some contain benzidine, a known cancer causer
GMOs	Nail polish, bubble bath, baby wipes, body wash, hair care	· Formaldehyde is a known cancer-causer · Linked to organ damage
*1,4-dioxane (PEG ingredients, and words that end in -eth (oleth, myreth, etc.))	Many conventionally grown foods such as apples, sugar beets, canola, and corn	· Linked to infertility, immune issues, organ damage, accelerated aging, GI and organ problems, and problems with insulin regulation

Ingredients to Avoid in Cosmetics and Personal Care Products

INGREDIENT	FOUND IN	HEALTH EFFECTS
Triclosan	Antibacterial products, including dish soap, some school supplies, and hand sanitizer	· Acts as an endocrine disruptor · Linked to increased allergies
Ethanolamines (DEA, MEA, TEA)	Soaps, shampoos, conditioner, baby wash, hand soaps	· Linked to liver tumors · Risk of contamination with nitrosamines (known cancer causers)
Sodium lauryl sulfate	Soaps, shampoos, bubble bath, body wash, facial soap, toothpaste, shaving cream	· Can be contaminated with different carcinogens · Linked to hair loss (in shampoo) · Highly irritating to the skin · May be a cause of canker sores (when in toothpaste)

INGREDIENT	FOUND IN	HEALTH EFFECTS
Mineral oil	Eye shadow, blush, lip gloss, lotions, hair products	• Inhibits skin's oil production • Can prevent the release of toxins through the skin • Possibly contaminated with cancer-causing hydrocarbons
Phthalates	Mascara and nail polish; can hide under the term *fragrance*	• Known as a probable human carcinogen • Act as endocrine disruptors • Linked to lower IQ with prenatal exposure
Fragrance	Hair care, cosmetics, baby wipes, body wash, bubble bath, nail polish, perfumes, body spray, hand sanitizer	• Can be made up of dozens to hundreds of chemicals, including some that act as endocrine disruptors • Linked to cancer and lower IQ • Considered to be a trade secret so individual ingredients are not required to be disclosed
Parabens (methylparaben, propylparaben, butylparaben, and ethylparaben)	Shampoo, deodorant, shave gels, moisturizers, lotions, sunscreens	• Act as endocrine disruptors • Have been found in biopsied breast cancer tumors
Methylisothiazolinone	Shampoos, baby wipes, sunscreens, moisturizers	• Strong allergen • May be toxic to the immune system • May be toxic to the brain and nervous system
*Formaldehyde releasers (quaternium-15, diazolidinyl urea, DMDM hydantoin, formalin)	Nail polish, bubble bath, baby wipes, body wash, hair care	• Formaldehyde is a known cancer causer • Linked to organ damage

Ingredients to Avoid in Cleaning Products

INGREDIENT	FOUND IN	HEALTH EFFECTS
Glycol ethers (most common type is 2-butoxyethanol)	Grease cutters and window cleaners (Simple Green, Formula 409, Windex, etc.)	• Liver cancer in lab animals • Exposure by inhalation and skin • Can go through rubber gloves
Alkylphenol ethoxylates (nonylphenol and octylphenol; nonoxynol)	Laundry detergents (may see them listed as "nonionic surfactants"), cleaning products, paint, hair care products, pesticides	• Mimics estrogen • Shown to multiply breast cancer cells in lab tests • May disrupt immune system • Bioaccumulates
Dye	All-purpose cleaners, window cleaners, toilet bowl cleaners, laundry detergents	• Term used to hide chemical info; not sure what ingredients it contains
Ethanolamines (DEA, MEA, TEA)	Degreasing formulas (Fantastik, Formula 409, Easy-Off, etc.), laundry detergents	• Possible contamination with nitrosamines (carcinogens) • Can trigger asthma attacks, even in those without asthma
Fragrance	Multipurpose cleaners, floor cleaners, laundry detergents, dryer sheets, window cleaners, dish soap, dusting sprays	• Endocrine disruption • Can be made up of hundreds, if not thousands of chemicals
Quaternary ammonium compounds (benzalkonium chloride)	Disinfecting sprays (Pine-Sol, Fantastik), fabric softeners and laundry detergents (Purex brand), oven cleaners, drain clog removers	• Can cause asthma and allergic reactions • Can cause severe skin burns and eye damage
Synthetic musk	Soap, cosmetics, laundry detergents, dryer sheets	• Enhances the effects of other toxic chemicals in products • Bioaccumulates

INGREDIENT	FOUND IN	HEALTH EFFECTS
Chlorinated phenol	Toilet bowl cleaners	· Toxic to the respiratory system
Diethylene glycol	Window cleaners	· Depresses the nervous system
Butyl cellusolve	All-purpose and window cleaners	· May damage liver, kidneys, bone marrow, and nervous system
Bleach	Products labeled "with bleach," chlorine bleach, countertop sprays, toilet bowl cleaners	· Can cause irritation in the eyes, mouth, lungs, and skin · Can be fatal if swallowed · Is corrosive internally and externally
Ammonia	Window cleaners, metal polishers, stainless steel and brass polishes, some all-purpose cleaners (especially those labeled "tough on grease")	· Moderate risk for respiratory concerns · Can cause dangerous, even deadly fumes, especially when mixed with bleach products

Notes

Chapter 1. Why *Slightly* Greener

1   *the list goes on:* "Flame Retardants," *Health & Education, National Institute of Environmental Health Sciences,* last reviewed March 5, 2020, https://www.niehs.nih.gov/health/topics/agents/flame _retardants/index.cfm.

2   *has skyrocketed:* Molly Miller, "Toxic Exposure: Chemicals are in Our Water, Food, Air, and Furniture," *University of California San Francisco Magazine,* June 22, 2017, https://www.ucsf.edu /news/2017/06/407416/toxic-exposure-chemicals-are-our-water-food-air-and-furniture.

3   *diabetes, and obesity:* "Obesity," Chronic Health Conditions, Centers for Disease Control and Prevention, last reviewed September 18, 2018, https://www.cdc.gov/healthyschools/obesity /facts.htm; Andrew Moore, "Increasing Rates of Allergies and Asthma," *American Academy of Allergy Asthma & Immunology,* last reviewed September 28, 2020, https://www.aaaai.org /conditions-and-treatments/library/allergy-library/prevalence-of-allergies-and-asthma; Jon Baio et. al., "Prevalence of Autism Spectrum Disorder Among Children Aged 8 Years," *Morbidity and Mortality Weekly Report* vol. 67(6); 1–23, Centers for Disease Control and Prevention, April 27, 2018, https://www.cdc.gov/mmwr/volumes/67/ss/ss6706a1.htm?s_cid=ss6706a1_w; "Key Statistics for Childhood Cancers," American Cancer Society, last reviewed August 24, 2020, https://www.cancer.org/cancer/cancer-in-children/key-statistics.html; "Diabetes," Fact Sheets, World Health Organization, June 8, 2020, https://www.who.int/news-room/fact-sheets/detail /diabetes.

4   *(TSCA) Inventory:* "EPA Releases First Major Update to Chemicals List in 40 Years," News Releases, United States Environmental Protection Agency, February 19, 2019, https://www.epa .gov/newsreleases/epa-releases-first-major-update-chemicals-list-40-years.

5   *according to scientists:* Flora Teoh, "The Most Popular Health Articles of 2018, a Scientific Credibility Review," Health Feedback, January 28, 2019, https://healthfeedback.org/the-most -popular-health-articles-of-2018-a-scientific-credibility-review/.

6   *skin is damaged:* "Skin Exposures and Effects," Workplace Safety & Health Topics, Centers for
      Disease Control and Prevention, last reviewed July 2, 2013, https://www.cdc.gov/niosh/topics
      /skin/default.html.

7   *is often unclear:* Ilona Silins and Johan Hogberg, "Combined Toxic Exposures and Human
      Health: Biomarkers of Exposure and Effect," *International Journal of Environmental Research and
      Public Health* 8, no. 3 (February 2011): 629–647, accessed via U.S. National Library of Medicine,
      https://www.ncbi.nlm.nih.gov/pmc/articles/PMC3083662/.

8   *experiencing at school:* James Greenblatt, "Dietary Influences on Behavioral Problems in
      Children," Integrative Medicine for Mental Health, June 7, 2017, https://www.immh.org/article
      -source/?category=Nutrition.

9   *eat a single one:* J. M. Peters et. al., "Processed Meats and Risk of Childhood Leukemia (California,
      USA)," *Cancer Causes Control* 5, no. 2 (1994): 195–202, accessed via PubMed, https://pubmed
      .ncbi.nlm.nih.gov/8167267/.

Chapter 2. Getting Started with the Slightly Greener Method

1   *and lower IQ:* "What Is Nieh Research Telling Us about Endocrine Disruptors?" Endocrine
      Disruptors Research, National Institute of Environmental Health Sciences, last reviewed May
      25, 2018, https://www.niehs.nih.gov/research/programs/endocrine/index.cfm.

2   *toys, and cosmetics:* T. T. Schug et. al., "Designing Endocrine Disruption Out of the Next
      Generation of Chemicals," *Green Chem* 15, no. 1 (January 2013): 181–198, accessed via U.S. National
      Library of Medicine, https://www.ncbi.nlm.nih.gov/pmc/articles/PMC4125359/.

3   *systems are developing:* Philippe Grandjean and Philip J. Landrigan, "Neurobehavioural Effects
      of Developmental Toxicity," *Lancet Neural* 13 (February 2014): 330–38, https://www.thelancet
      .com/pdfs/journals/laneur/PIIS1474-4422(13)70278-3.pdf; "Prenatal Exposure to Common
      Chemicals Linked to Lower IQ," Child and Adolescent Health, Environmental Health, Maternal
      and Reproductive Health, Columbia Mailman School of Public Health, December 10, 2014,
      https://www.mailman.columbia.edu/public-health-now/news/prenatal-exposure-common
      -chemicals-linked-lower-iq.

4   *regulation and weight:* San-Nan Yang et. al., "The Effects of Environmental Toxins on Allergic
      Inflammation," *Allergy Asthma Immunol Research* 6, no. 6 (October 2014): 478–484, accessed via
      U.S. National Library of Medicine, https://www.ncbi.nlm.nih.gov/pmc/articles/PMC4214967/;
      "Chemical Present in Clear Plastics Can Impair Learning and Cause Disease," Yale News,
      March 28, 2005, https://news.yale.edu/2005/03/28/chemical-present-clear-plastics-can-impair
      -learning-and-cause-disease.

5   *feeling of being full:* Wendee Holtcamp, "Obesogens: An Environmental Link to Obesity,"
      Environmental Health Perspectives 120, no. 20 (February 2012): a62-a68, accessed via U.S. National
      Library of Medicine, https://www.ncbi.nlm.nih.gov/pmc/articles/PMC3279464/; Philippa D.
      Darbre, "Endocrine Disruptors and Obesity," *Current Obesity Reports* 6, no. 1 (February 2017): 18–

27, accessed via U.S. National Library of Medicine, https://www.ncbi.nlm.nih.gov/pmc/articles /PMC5359373/.

6   *can cause cancer:* "Cancer-causing Substances in the Environment," National Cancer Institute, updated December 28, 2018, https://www.cancer.gov/about-cancer/causes-prevention/risk /substances.

7   *exacerbate allergies:* S. W. P. Wijnhoven et. al., "Allergens in Consumer Products," RIVM Report 320025001, National Institute for Public Health and the Environment, 2008, https://www.rivm .nl/bibliotheek/rapporten/320025001.pdf; Jane A. Hoppin et. al., "Pesticides are Associated with Allergic and Non-Allergic Wheezing among Male Farmers," *Environmental Health Perspectives* 125, no.4 (July 2016): 535–543, accessed via U.S. National Library of Medicine, https://www.ncbi .nlm.nih.gov/pmc/articles/PMC5381985/.

8   *are far greater:* William W. Au, "Susceptibility of Children to Environmental Toxic Substances," *International Journal of Hygiene and Environmental Health* 205, no.6 (October 2002): 501–3, accessed via PubMed, https://www.ncbi.nlm.nih.gov/pubmed/12455272.

9   *than an adult does:* Philip J. Ladrigan and Lynn R. Goldman, "Children's Vulnerability to Toxic Chemicals: A Challenge and Opportunity to Strengthen Health and Environmental Policy," *Health Affairs* 30, no.5, published online May 1, 2011, https://www.healthaffairs.org/doi /full/10.1377/hlthaff.2011.0151.

10   *lifelong impairments:* Travis Madsen and Elizabeth Hitchcock, "Growing Up Toxic: Chemical Exposures and Increases in Developmental Disease," U.S. Public Interest Research Group Education Fund, March 2011, https://frontiergroup.org/sites/default/files/reports/Growing-Up -Toxic-Update_us.pdf.

11   *exposure in infancy:* Jason R. Cannon and J. Timothy Greenamyre, "The Role of Environmental Exposures in Neurodegeneration and Neurodegenerative Diseases," *Toxicological Sciences* 124, no.2: 225–250, published online September 13, 2011, accessed via U.S. National Library of Medicine, https://www.ncbi.nlm.nih.gov/pmc/articles/PMC3216414/.

12   *newborns tested:* "Body Burden: The Pollution in Newborns," Environmental Working Group, July 14, 2005, https://www.ewg.org/research/body-burden-pollution-newborns.

13   *EPA's Science Advisory Board:* "SAB Review of EPA's Draft Risk Assessment of the Potential Human Health Effects Associated with PFOA and Its Salts," U.S. Environmental Protection Agency, May 30, 2006, accessed via National Service Center for Environmental Publications, https://nepis.epa.gov/Exe/ZyPURL.cgi?Dockey=901S0J00.TXT.

14   *diagnosed learning disorder:* "National Report Sheds Light on Struggles of Students with Learning Disabilities and How Parents Educators, Physicians, and Policymakers Can Help," National Center for Learning Disabilities, May 2, 2017, https://ncld.org/news/newsroom/the-state-of-ld -understanding-the-1-in-5.

15   *since 1980:* "Obesity," Centers for Disease Control and Prevention.

16   *or hay fever:* "Why kids born in the U.S. have more allergies, asthma," Advisory Board, May 1,

2013, https://www.advisory.com/daily-briefing/2013/05/01/why-kids-born-in-the-us-have-more-allergies-asthma#:.

17   *1997 and 2011:* Kristen D. Jackson et. al., "Trends in Allergic Conditions Among Children: United States 1997–2011," *National Center for Health Statistics Data Brief* no. 121, May 2013, accessed via Centers for Disease Control and Prevention, https://www.cdc.gov/nchs/data/databriefs/db121.pdf.

18   *worsening asthma symptoms:* Code of Federal Regulations Title 21—Food and Drugs, revised as of April 1, 2019, accessed via U.S. Department of Health & Human Services, https://www.accessdata.fda.gov/scripts/cdrh/cfdocs/cfcfr/CFRSearch.cfm?fr=201.20.

19   *learning and cognition:* L. Eugene Arnold et. al., "Artificial Food Colors and Attention-Deficit/Hyperactivity Symptoms: Conclusions to Dye for," *Neurotherapeutics* vol. 9(3): 599–609, published online August 3, 2012, accessed via U.S. National Library of Medicine, https://www.ncbi.nlm.nih.gov/pmc/articles/PMC3441937/; Wafaa M. Abdel Moneim et. al., "Monosodium Glutamate Affects Cognitive Functions in Male Albino Rats," *Egyptian Journal of Forensic Sciences* vol. 8(9), published online January 26, 2018, accessed via Springer Link, https://link.springer.com/article/10.1186/s41935-018-0038-x; Mj Khoshnoud et. al., "Effects of sodium benzoate, a commonly used food preservative, on learning, memory, and oxidative stress in brain of mice," *Journal of Biochemical and Molecular Toxicology* vol.32(2), December 2017, accessed via Research Gate, https://www.researchgate.net/publication/321855885_Effects_of_sodium_benzoate_a_commonly_used_food_preservative_on_learning_memory_and_oxidative_stress_in_brain_of_mice.

20   *childhood cancer and leukemia:* Peters et. al., "Processed Meats," 195–202.

Chapter 3. The Power of Starting Small

1   *your long-term health:* "Reducing the Impact of Hazardous Chemicals on Public Health: What Is Known and What Can Be Done to Reduce It?" Green Facts, last updated October 15, 2018, https://www.greenfacts.org/en/chemicals-public-health/index.htm.

2   *buildup in your body:* Miller, "Toxic Exposure."

3   *almost 60 percent!:* Carly Hyland et. al., "Organic Diet Intervention Significantly Reduces Urinary Pesticide Levels in U.S. Children and Adults," *Environmental Research* vol. 171 (April 2019): 568–574, accessed via Science Direct, https://www.sciencedirect.com/science/article/pii/S0013935119300246?via%3Dihub.

4   *diseases and illnesses:* Nicole Bijlsma et. al., "Environmental Chemical Assessment in Clinical Practice: Unveiling the Elephant in the Room," *International Journal of Environmental Research and Public Health* vol. 13(2): 181, published online February 2, 2016, accessed via U.S. National Library of Medicine, https://www.ncbi.nlm.nih.gov/pmc/articles/PMC4772201/.

5   *average of 35 percent:* Kim G. Harley et. al., "Reducing Phthalate, Paraben, and Phenol Exposure from Personal Care Products in Adolescent Girls: Finding HERMOSA Intervention Study,

Environmental Health Perspectives vol. 124(10), published online October 1, 2016, https://ehp.niehs .nih.gov/doi/10.1289/ehp.1510514.

6   *being heavily exposed:* Bruce P. Lanphear and Linda S. Birnbaum, "Low-Level Toxicity of Chemicals: No Acceptable Levels?" *PLOS Biology* vol. 15(12): e2003066, published online December 19, 2017, accessed via U.S. National Library of Medicine, https://www.ncbi.nlm.nih .gov/pmc/articles/PMC5736171/.

7   *exacerbated by them:* "Health Effects of Chemical Exposure," Agency for Toxic Substances and Disease Registry, https://www.atsdr.cdc.gov/emes/public/docs/health%20effects%20of%20 chemical%20exposure%20fs.pdf.

8   *remove harmful substances:* "Introduction to Biotransformation," Environmental Health & Toxicology Information, U.S. National Library of Medicine, accessed November 2020, https:// toxtutor.nlm.nih.gov/12–001.html.

9   *located in the liver:* Donald R. Buhler and David E. Williams, "The Role of Biotransformation in the Toxicity of Chemicals," *Aquatic Toxicology* vol. 11 (1998): 19–28, accessed via Science Direct, https://www.sciencedirect.com/science/article/abs/pii/0166445X88900045.

10   *and nutritional status:* Wayne L. Sodano and Ron Grisanti, "The Physiology and Biochemisty of Biotransformation/Detoxification (The Phases of Detoxification)," Functional Medicine Diagnostic Medicine Training Program, Function Medicine University, 2010, http://www .functionalmedicineuniversity.com/fdmt551aphysiobiodetoxig.pdf.

11   *disrupted in some way:* Maya E. Kotas and Ruslan Medzhitov, "Homeostasis, Inflammation, and Disease Susceptibility," *Cell* vol. 160(5): 816–827, published online February 26, 2015, accessed via U.S. National Library of Medicine, https://www.ncbi.nlm.nih.gov/pmc/articles/PMC4369762/.

12   *dysregulated and fail:* Dickson Thom et. al., *Bioregulatory Medicine: An Innovative Holistic Approach to Self-Healing* (White River Junction, Vermont: Chelsea Green Publishing, 2018), 3.

13   *at any given time:* "Body Burden," Science Direct, https://www.sciencedirect.com/topics /medicine-and-dentistry/body-burden.

14   *urine or feces:* Barbara Scott Murdock, "Tracking Toxins," *EMBO Reports* vol. 6(8): 701–705, published online August 6, 2005, accessed via U.S. National Library of Medicine, https://www .ncbi.nlm.nih.gov/pmc/articles/PMC1369152/.

15   *exit the body:* "Pesticide Half-life: Topic Fact Sheet," National Pesticide Information Center, last reviewed May 2015, http://npic.orst.edu/factsheets/half-life.html.

16   *increase body burden:* "Bioaccumulation," Science Direct, https://www.sciencedirect.com/topics /pharmacology-toxicology-and-pharmaceutical-science/bioaccumulation.

17   *environment whenever possible:* Robert Scheuplein et. al., "Differential Sensitivity of Children and Adults to Chemical Toxicity: I. Biological Basis," *Regular Toxicology and Pharmacology* vol.35(3): 429–447, June 2002, accessed via Science Direct, https://www.sciencedirect.com/science/article /abs/pii/S0273230002915588.

18   *measure and trace:* Daniel Goleman, "Our Bodies' Chemical Burden: Little Doses Matter a Lot,"

Pollution in People, Environmental Working Group, April 26, 2010, https://www.ewg.org/kid-safe-chemicals-act-blog/2010/04/our-bodies%E2%80%99-chemical-burden-little-doses-matter-a-lot/.

19　*issues in children:* Tye E. Arbuckle et. al., "Bisphenol a, Phthalates and Lead and Learning and Behavorial Problems in Canadian Children 6–11 Years of Age: CHMS 2007–2009," *Neurotoxicology* vol. 54: 89–98, published online March 26, 2016, accessed via Science Direct, https://www.sciencedirect.com/science/article/pii/S0161813X16300365.

20　*in the freezer:* Hoa H. Le et. al., "Bisphenol a Is Released from Polycarbonate Drinking Bottles and Mimics the Neurotoxic Actions of Estrogen in Developing Cerebellar Neurons," *Toxicology Letters* 176, no. 2: 149–156, published online November 19, 2007, accessed via U.S. National Library of Medicine, https://www.ncbi.nlm.nih.gov/pmc/articles/PMC2254523/.

21　*to ADHD in children:* Maryse F. Bouchard et. al., "Attention Deficit/Hyperactivity Disorder and Urinary Metabolites of Organophosphate Pesticides in U.S. Children 8–15 Years," *Pediatrics* 125, no.6: e1270-e1277, published online May 17, 2010, accessed via U.S. National Library of Medicine, https://www.ncbi.nlm.nih.gov/pmc/articles/PMC3706632/.

22　*loss of 16.9 million IQ points:* David C. Bellinger, "A Strategy for Comparing the Contributions of Environmental Chemicals and Other Risk Factors to Neurodevelopment of Children," *Environmental Health Perspectives* 120, no. 4 (April 2012): 501–7, https://doi.org/10.1289/ehp.1104170.

23　*before being consumed:* Bonnie Bruce et. al., "A Diet High in Whole and Unrefined Foods Favorably Alters Lipids, Antioxidant Defenses, and Colon Function," *Journal of the American College of Nutrition* 19, no. 1 (2000): 61–67, http://gethealthygethot.com/61.pdf.

24　*(and nervous system):* "Health Effects and Chemical of Concern," Campaign for Safe Cosmetics, accessed November 2020 http://www.safecosmetics.org/fragrance-disclosure/learn-more/health-effects-chemical-concern/.

25　*infections in infants:* "Air Fresheners Can Make Mothers and Babies Ill," Avon Longitudinal Study of Parents and Children, University of Bristol, October 19, 2004, https://www.bristol.ac.uk/alspac/news/2004/75.html.

26　*when burned:* Tomasz Olszowski and Andrzej Klos, "The Impact of Candle Burning During All Saints' Day Ceremonies on Ambient Alkyl-Substituted Benzene Concentrations," *Bulletin of Environmental Contamination and Toxicology* 91, no. 5 (2013): 588–594, https://www.ncbi.nlm.nih.gov/pmc/articles/PMC3824304/ .

27　*weight gain, and cancer:* "Potentially Harmful Chemicals Widespread in Household Dust," Milken Institute School of Public Health at the George Washington University, September 14, 2016, https://publichealth.gwu.edu/content/potentially-harmful-chemicals-widespread-household-dust.

28　*(and lower IQ):* Haotian Wu et. al., "Parental Contributions to Early Embryo Development: Influences of Urinary Phthalate and Phthalate Alternatives among Couples Undergoing Ivf Treatment," *Human Reproduction* 32, no.1: 65–75, published online December 16, 2016, https://

academic.oup.com/humrep/article/32/1/65/2631391; Xiyan Mu et. al., "New Insights into the Mechanism of Phthalate-Induced Developmental Effects," *Environmental Pollution* 241: 674–683, published online June 11, 2018, accessed via Science Direct, https://www.sciencedirect.com /science/article/pii/S0269749117348571; Claude Monneret, "What Is an Endocrine Disruptor," *Comptes Rendus Biologies* 340, no. 9–10: 403–405, published online November 7, 2017, accessed via Science Direct, https://www.sciencedirect.com/science/article/pii/S1631069117301257; A. Broe et. al., "Association between Use of Phthalate-Containing Medication and Semen Quality among Men in Couples Referred for Assisted Reproduction," *Human Reproduction* 33, no. 3 (March 2018): 503–511, https://academic.oup.com/humrep/article/33/3/503/4841815; Eva M. Tanner et. al., "Early Prenatal Exposure to Suspected Endocrine Disruptor Mixtures Is Associated with Lower IQ at Age Seven," *Environmental International* 134: 105185, published online October 24, 2019, accessed via Science Direct, https://www.sciencedirect.com/science/article/pii /S0160412019314011; Ling-Chuan Guo et. al., "Human Sex Hormone Disrupting Effects of New Flame Retardants and Their Interactions with Polychlorinated Biphenyls, Polybrominated Diphenyl Ethers, a Case Study in South China," *Environmental Science & Technology* 52, no. 23 (2018): 13935–13941, accessed via ACS Publications, https://pubs.acs.org/doi/abs/10.1021/acs .est.8b01540; Shannon T. Lipscomb et. al., "Cross-sectional study of social behaviors in preschool children and exposure to flame retardants," *Environmental Health* 16 (2017), accessed via BMC, https://ehjournal.biomedcentral.com/articles/10.1186/s12940-017-0224-6; Michelle Kira Lee and Bruce Blumberg, "Transgenerational effects of obesogens," *Basic & Clinical Pharmocology & Toxicology* 125, not. S3 (August 2019): 44–57, accessed via Wiley Online Library, https:// onlinelibrary.wiley.com/doi/full/10.1111/bcpt.13214; Mandana Ghisari et. al., "Polymorphism in Xenobiotic and Estrogen Metabolizing Genes, Exposure to Perfluorinated Compounds and Subsequent Breast Cancer Risk," *Environmental Research* 154: 325–333, published online February 2, 2017, accessed via Science Direct, https://www.sciencedirect.com/science/article/abs/pii /S0013935116305266; "Immunotoxicity Associated with Exposure to Perfluorooctanoic Acid (PFOA) or Perfluorooctane Sulfate (PFOS), National Toxicology Program," U.S. Dept. of Health and Human Services, last updated January 24, 2020, https://ntp.niehs.nih.gov/whatwestudy /assessments/noncancer/completed/pfoa/index.html; Samuel Caito et. al., "Developmental Neurotoxicity of Lead," in *Neurotoxicity of Metals* vol. 18, ed. M. Aschner (Springer, 2017), 3–12, https://link.springer.com/chapter/10.1007/978-3-319-60189-2_1.

Chapter 4. Learn to Read Ingredients, Not Labels

1   *average grocery store:* Andrew F. Smith, *Food in America: The Past, Present, and Future of Food, Farming, and the Family Meal*, vol. 1 (ABC-CLIO, 2017).

2   *to over fifty thousand:* Michael Ruhlman, *Grocery: The Buying and Selling of Food in America,* (New York: Abrams Press, 2017), 29–30.

3   *organic farming movement:* "History of Organic Farming in the United States," Sustainable

Agriculture Research and Education (SARE), accessed November 2020, https://www.sare.org/Learning-Center/Bulletins/Transitioning-to-Organic-Production/Text-Version/History-of-Organic-Farming-in-the-United-States.

4   *today as organic farming:* Tom Philpott, "Reviving a Much-Cited, Little-Read Sustainable-Ag Masterpiece," *Grist*, March 2, 2007, https://grist.org/article/soil/.

5   *less than one percent!:* Kristen Bialik and Kristi Walker, "Organic Farming Is on The Rise in The U.S.," Pew Research Center, January 10, 2019, https://www.pewresearch.org/fact-tank/2019/01/10/organic-farming-is-on-the-rise-in-the-u-s/.

6   *oversees the USDA organic label:* "Rules and Regulations," National Organic Standards Board, Agricultural Marketing Service, accessed November 2020, https://www.ams.usda.gov/rules-regulations/organic/nosb; Karen Asp, "Is the Organic Label as Valuable as You Thought?" Hunter College New York City Food Policy Center, December 6, 2018, https://www.nycfoodpolicy.org/is-the-organic-label-as-valuable-as-you-thought/.

7   *USDA's Agricultural Marketing Service:* Miles McEvoy, "Organic 101: Understanding the Made with Organic*** Label," U.S. Department of Agriculture, February 21, 2017, https://www.usda.gov/media/blog/2014/05/16/organic-101-understanding-made-organic-label.

8   *at every single step:* "4 Categories of Organic Product Labels," Global Organics, March 29, 2016, https://www.global-organics.com/post.php?s=2016-03-29-4-categories-of-organic-product-labels.

9   *produced and processed:* "Labeling Organic Products," USDA National Organic Program/Agricultural Marketing Service, December 2016, https://www.ams.usda.gov/sites/default/files/media/Labeling%20Organic%20Products.pdf.

10   *what they signify:* "Pesticides and Human Health," Californians for Pesticide Reform, accessed November 2020, https://www.pesticidereform.org/pesticides-human-health/; "Organic Labeling Standards," Agricultural Marketing Service, U.S. Department of Agriculture, accessed November 2020, https://www.ams.usda.gov/grades-standards/organic-labeling-standards.

11   *Prohibited Substances:* Miles McEvoy, "Organic 101: Allowed and Prohibited Substances," U.S. Department of Agriculture, October 27, 2020, https://www.usda.gov/media/blog/2012/01/25/organic-101-allowed-and-prohibited-substances.

12   *the following criteria:* "Evaluation Criteria for Allowed and Prohibited Substances, Methods, and Ingredients," The National List of Allowed and Prohibited Substances, accessed via Electronic Code of Federal Regulations, November 2020, https://www.ecfr.gov/cgi-bin/text-idx?c=ecfr&SID=9874504b6f1025eb0e6b67cadf9d3b40&rgn=div6&view=text&node=7:3.1.1.9.32.7&idno=7#se7.3.205_1600.

13   *"and blueberries":* McEvoy, "Organic 101: Understanding the Made with Organic *** Label."

14   *from the USDA:* "Mandatory Labeling Requirements," USDA, August 22, 2016, https://www.ams.usda.gov/sites/default/files/media/USDA%20Grademarked%20Product%20Label%20Submission%20Checklist.pdf.

15   *the outdoor area:* ibid.

16   *"fatty acids.":* ibid.

17   *consume enough of them:* Freydis Hjalmarsdottir, "17 Science-Based Benefits of Omega-3 Fatty Acids," *Healthline,* October 15, 2018, https://www.healthline.com/nutrition/17-health-benefits -of-omega-3#section5.

18   *of the flocks:* "Mandatory Labeling Requirements," USDA.

19   *or other drugs:* Laura J. Martin, "Are Some Eggs Safer than Others?" WebMD, August 25, 2010, https://www.webmd.com/food-recipes/features/egg-types-benefits-facts#2.

20   *on the label:* "Mandatory Labeling Requirements," USDA.

21   *organic food regularly:* "Study: 82% of U.S. Households Buy Organic Food Regularly," Ag Web, March 24, 2017, https://www.agweb.com/article/study-82-of-us-households-buy-organic-food -regularly-NAA-nate-birt.

22   *pests and weeds:* "Organic vs. Conventional Farming," Rodale Institute, accessed November 2020, https://rodaleinstitute.org/why-organic/organic-basics/organic-vs-conventional/.

23   *after it is washed:* EWG Science Team, "EWG's 2020 Shopper's Guide to Pesticides in Produce," Environmental Working Group, March 25, 2020, https://www.ewg.org/foodnews/summary.php.

24   *at particular risk:* "Pesticide Exposures," National Center for Environmental Health, updated April 12, 2019, accessed via Centers for Disease Control and Prevention website, https:// ephtracking.cdc.gov/showPesticidesHealth.

25   *urine and blood:* Yu-Han Chiu et. al., "Comparison of questionnaire-based estimation of pesticide residue intake from fruits and vegetables with urinary concentrations of pesticide biomarkers," *Journal of Exposure Science and Environmental Epidemiology* 28, no. 1: 31–39, published online September 20, 2017, accessed via U.S. National Library of Medicine, https://www.ncbi .nlm.nih.gov/pmc/articles/PMC5734986/.

26   *and other organs:* "Long-term Health Effects of Pesticides," in *A Community Guide to Environmental Health,* by Jeff Conant and Pam Fadem (Berkeley, CA: Hesperian, 2012), 261–263, accessed via Hesperian Health Guides website, https://en.hesperian.org/hhg/A_Community_Guide_to _Environmental_Health:Long-term_Health_Effects_of_Pesticides.

27   *rates of ADHD:* Virginia Rush et. al., "Seven-Year Neurodevelopmental Scores and Prenatal Exposure to Chlorpyrifos, a Common Agricultural Pesticide," *Environmental Health Perspectives* 119, no. 8 (August 1, 2018): 1196–1201, https://ehp.niehs.nih.gov/doi/10.1289/ehp.1003160; Bouchard et. al., "Attention-Deficit/Hyperactivity Disorder and Urinary Metabolites of Organophosphate Pesticides"; Virginia A. Rauh et. al., "Impact of Prenatal Chlorpyrifos Exposure on Neurodevelopment in the First 3 Years of Life Among Inner-City Children," *Pediatrics* 118, no.6 (December 2006): e1845-e1859, https://pediatrics.aappublications.org/content/118/6/e1845.

28   *them out too:* Rauh, "Impact of Prenatal Chlorpyrifos Exposure on Neurodevelopment in the First 3 Years of Life Among Inner-City Children."; B. Gomez-Gimenez et. al., "Developmental Exposure to Pesticides Alters Motor Activity and Coordination in Rats: Sex Differences and Underlying Mechanisms," *Neurotoxicity Research* 33 (2018): 247–258, accessed via Springer Link,

https://link.springer.com/article/10.1007%2Fs12640-017-9823-9; Belen Gomez-Gimenez et. al., "Sex-dependent effects of developmental exposure to different pesticides on spatial learning. The rose of induced neuroinflammation in the hippocampus," *Food and Chemical Toxicology* 99: 135–148, published online November 29, 2016, accessed via Science Direct, https://www.sciencedirect.com/science/article/pii/S0278691516304458?via%3Dihub.

29   *to what adults eat:* "Fast Facts about Health Risks of Pesticides in Food," Center for Ecogenetic and Environmental Health, University of Washington School of Public Health, January 2013, https://depts.washington.edu/ceeh/downloads/FF_Pesticides.pdf.

30   *"during early childhood":* "Overexposed: Organophosphate Insecticides in Children's Food," Environmental Working Group, January 29, 1998, https://www.ewg.org/research/overexposed-organophosphate-insecticides-childrens-food.

31   *pesticides in our bodies:* Asa Bradman et. al., "Effect of Organic Diet Intervention on Pesticide Exposures in Young Children Living in Low-Income Urban and Agricultural Communities," *Environmental Health Perspectives* 123, no.10 (October 2015): 1086–1093, https://ehp.niehs.nih.gov/doi/10.1289/ehp.1408660.

32   *versus non-organic foods:* Michelle Brandt, "Little evidence of health benefits from organic foods, study finds," Stanford Medicine News Center, September 2012, https://med.stanford.edu/news/all-news/2012/09/little-evidence-of-health-benefits-from-organic-foods-study-finds.html.

33   *than nonorganic:* Marcin Baranski et. al., "Higher Antioxidant and Lower Cadmium Concentrations and Lower Incidence of Pesticide Residues in Organically Grown Crops; a Systematic Literature Review and Meta-Analyses," *British Journal of Nutrition* 112, no. 5 (September 2014): 794–811, accessed via PubMed, https://www.ncbi.nlm.nih.gov/pubmed/24968103.

34   *or even cancer:* "Flavanols," Science Direct, accessed November 2020, https://www.sciencedirect.com/topics/neuroscience/flavonols.

35   *and overall health:* "The 411 on Flavanoids," Nutritious Life, accessed November 2020, https://nutritiouslife.com/eat-empowered/flavanols-cocoa-health-benefits/.

36   *more omega-3 fatty acids:* Allison Aubrey, "Is Organic More Nutritious? New Study Adds to the Evidence," *NPR,* February 18, 2016, https://www.npr.org/sections/thesalt/2016/02/18/467136329/is-organic-more-nutritious-new-study-adds-to-the-evidence.

37   *The Clean 15:* "Clean 15: EWG's 2020 Shopper's Guide to Pesticides in Produce," Environmental Working Group, accessed November 2020, https://www.ewg.org/foodnews/clean-fifteen.php.

38   *The Dirty Dozen:* "Dirty Dozen: EWG's 2020 Shopper's Guide to Pesticides in Produce," Environmental Working Group, accessed November 2020, https://www.ewg.org/foodnews/dirty-dozen.php.

39   *wholesale market:* Luke Denne and Tiffany Foxcraft, " 'People Are Being Duped': CBC exposes homegrown lies at farmers markets," *CBC News,* September 29, 2017, https://www.cbc.ca/news/business/farmers-markets-lies-marketplace-1.4306231.

40 *(not organic) farms:* Tara Parker-Pope, "Deception at the Farmer's Market," *The New York Times,* September 24, 2010, https://well.blogs.nytimes.com/2010/09/24/deception-at-the-farmers -market.

41 *and no GMOs:* Andrea Rock, "Peeling Back the 'Natural' Food Label," *Consumer Reports,* January 27, 2016, https://www.consumerreports.org/food-safety/peeling-back-the-natural-food-label/; Consumer Reports Media Room, "Consumer Reports Survey Show 73 Percent of Consumers Look for 'Natural' Labels at Grocery Stores—and Many are Unwittingly Misled," *Consumer Reports,* May, 10, 2016, https://www.washingtonpost.com/news/wonk/wp/2014/06/24/the -word-natural-helps-sell-40-billion-worth-of-food-in-the-u-s-every-year-and-the-label-means -nothing/?utm_term=.55e8379927c9.

42 *(by the FDA):* "Why We Rate Food-Label Seals & Claims," Consumer Report's Guide to Food Labels, *Consumer Reports,* 2020, https://www.consumerreports.org/food-labels/seals-and-claims.

43 *sales in 2013:* Roberto A. Ferdman, "The Word 'Natural' Helps Sell $40 Billion Worth of Food in the U.S. Every Year—and the Label Means Nothing, " *The Washington Post,* June 24, 2014, https:// www.washingtonpost.com/news/wonk/wp/2014/06/24/the-word-natural-helps-sell-40-billion -worth-of-food-in-the-u-s-every-year-and-the-label-means-nothing/?utm_term=.55e8379927c9.

44 *"pesticide-free" labels:* Jessica Branch, "What Do You Really Get When You Buy Organic?" *Consumer Reports,* September 12, 2019, https://www.consumerreports.org/organic-foods/what -do-you-really-get-when-you-buy-organic/.

45 *is about six:* "How Much Is Too Much?" Sugar Science, University of California San Francisco, accessed November 2020, https://sugarscience.ucsf.edu/the-growing-concern-of -overconsumption.html#.XuhRlZ5Kjlw.

46 *as much as possible:* Eun Ha Seo et. al., "Association between Total Sugar Intake and Metabolic Syndrome in Middle-Aged Korean Men and Women," *Nutrients* 11, no. 9: 2042, published online September 1, 2019, accessed via U.S. National Library of Medicine, https://www.ncbi.nlm .nih.gov/pmc/articles/PMC6769797/; Chiadi E. Ndumele, "Obesity, Sugar, and Heart Health," Wellness and Prevention, Johns Hopkins Medicine, accessed November 2020, https://www .hopkinsmedicine.org/health/wellness-and-prevention/obesity-sugar-and-heart-health; Nour Makarem et. al., "Consumption of Sugars, Sugary Foods, and Sugary Beverages in Relation to Cancer Risk: A Systematic Review of Longitudinal Studies," *Annual Review Nutrition* 38 (August 2018): 17–39, accessed via PubMed, https://pubmed.ncbi.nlm.nih.gov/29801420/.

47 *from heart disease:* Quanhe Yang et. al., "Added Sugar Intake and Cardiovascular Diseases Mortality Among U.S. Adults," *JAMA Internal Medicine* 174, no. 4 (2014): 516–524, accessed via JAMA Network, https://jamanetwork.com/journals/jamainternalmedicine/fullarticle/1819573.

48 *and stroke risk:* James J. DiNicolantonio and Sean C. Lucan, "The Wrong White Crystals: Not Salt but Sugar as Aetiological in Hypertension and Cardiometabolic Disease," *Open Heart* 1, no.1: e000167, published online November 3, 2014, accessed via U.S. National Library of Medicine, https://www.ncbi.nlm.nih.gov/pmc/articles/PMC4336865/; "The Sweet Danger of

Sugar," Harvard Health Publishing, Harvard Medical School, published May 2017, updated November 5, 2019, https://www.health.harvard.edu/heart-health/the-sweet-danger-of-sugar; Metin Basaranoglu et. al., "Carbohydrate intake and nonalcoholic fatty liver disease: fructose as a weapon of mass destruction," *Hepatobiliary Surgery and Nutrition* 4, no.2 (April 2015): 109–116, accessed via U.S. National Library of Medicine, https://www.ncbi.nlm.nih.gov/pmc/articles /PMC4405421/.

Chapter 5. "Safe" Ingredients to Avoid

1   *in this country:* U.S. Burden of Disease Collaborators, "The State of U.S. Health, 1990–2016: Burden of Diseases, Injuries, and Risk Factors Among U.S. States," *JAMA* 319, no.14 (April 2018): 1444–1472, accessed via JAMA Network, https://jamanetwork.com/journals/jama /fullarticle/2678018?utm_campaign=articlePDF&utm_medium=articlePDFlink&utm_source =articlePDF&utm_content=jama.2018.0158.

2   *taste, or appearance:* Leonardo Trasande et. al., "Food Additives and Child Health," *Pediatrics* 142, no. 2 (August 2018): e20181408, accessed via AAP News & Journals Gateway, https://pediatrics .aappublications.org/content/142/2/e20181408.

3   *"recognize as food":* Michael Pollan, *Food Rules: An Eater's Manual,* (New York: Penguin Books, 2009), 148.

4   *contained phthalates:* ibid.

5   *the possible sources:* Ami Zota et. al., "Recent Fast Food Consumption and Bispheno A and Phthalates Exposures among the U.S. Population in NHANES, 2003–2010," *Environmental Health Perspectives* 124, no. 10 (October 2016): 1521–1528, https://ehp.niehs.nih.gov/doi/10.1289 /ehp.1510803.

6   *chicken nugget (1963):* Maryn Mckenna, "The Father of the Chicken Nugget," *Slate,* December 28, 2012, https://slate.com/human-interest/2012/12/robert-c-baker-the-man-who-invented-chicken -nuggets.html.

7   *corn syrup (1967):* Kay Parker et. al., "High Fructose Corn Syrup: Production, Uses and Public Health Concerns," *Biotechnology and Molecular Biology Review* 5, no. 5 (December 2010): 71–78, https://academicjournals.org/article/article1380113250_Parker%20et%20al.pdf.

8   *and Tang (1959):* Matt Blitz, "How NASA Made Tang Cool," *Food & Wine,* May 18, 2017, https:// www.foodandwine.com/lifestyle/how-nasa-made-tang-cool.

9   *introduction of Tab:* Laura M. Holson, "Where Has All the Tab Gone? A Shortage Panics Fans," *The New York Times,* October 17, 2018, https://www.nytimes.com/2018/10/17/business/tab -shortage-coca-cola.html.

10   *as well as Pringles:* Jeremy Caplan, "The Man Buried in a Pringles Can," *TIME,* June 4, 2008, http://content.time.com/time/business/article/0,8599,1811730,00.html.

11   *and Gatorade:* Daniel Roberts and Kacy Burdette, "The history of an iconic sports beverage: Gatorade turns 50," *Fortune,* October 1, 2015, https://fortune.com/2015/10/01/gatorade-turns-50/.

12 *for eleven years:* Remy Melina, "Why Were Red M&M's Discontinued for a Decade?" *Live Science,* February 10, 2011, https://www.livescience.com/33017-why-were-red-mms-discontinued-for-a -decade.html.

13 *in a school lunch:* Mary Thornton and Martin Schram, "U.S. Holds the Ketchup in Schools," *The Washington Post,* September 26, 1981, https://www.washingtonpost.com/archive/politics /1981/09/26/us-holds-the-ketchup-in-schools/9ffd029a-17f5–4e8c-ab91–1348a44773ee/.

14 *caloric sweeteners:* George A. Bray et. al., "Consumption of High-Fructose Corn Syrup in Beverages May Play a Role in the Epidemic of Obesity," *American Journal of Clinical Nutrition* 79, no. 4 (April 2004): 537–543, accessed via Oxford Academic, https://academic.oup.com/ajcn /article/79/4/537/4690128.

15 *standard nutrition labeling:* "History of Nutrition Labeling," in *Front-of-Package Nutrition Rating Systems and Symbols: Phase I Report,* edited by C.S. Boon et. al., (Washington D.C.: National Academies Press, 2010), accessed via U.S. National Library of Medicine.

16 *added to processed food:* Thomas G. Neltner et. al., "Navigating the U.S. Food Additive Regulatory Program," *Comprehensive Reviews in Food Science and Food Safety* 10, no. 6 (November 2011): 342– 368, accessed via Wiley Online Library, https://onlinelibrary.wiley.com/doi/full/10.1111/j.1541 -4337.2011.00166.x.

17 *effects are unknown:* Leonardo Trasande et. al., "Food Additives and Child Health," *Pediatrics* 142, no. 2 (August 2018): e20181408, accessed via American Academy of Pediatrics Gateway, https:// pediatrics.aappublications.org/content/142/2/e20181408.

18 *about additives used:* Thomas N. Neltner et. al., "Navigating the U.S. Food Additive Regulatory Program," *Comprehensive Reviews in Food Science and Food Safety* 10, not. 6 (2011): 342–368, accessed via Wiley Online Library, https://onlinelibrary.wiley.com/doi/full/10.1111/j.1541 -4337.2011.00166.x; Erin Quinn and Chris Young, "Why the FDA Doesn't Really Know What's in Your Food," *The Center for Public Integrity,* April 24, 2015, https://publicintegrity.org/politics /why-the-fda-doesnt-really-know-whats-in-your-food/.

19 *to be safe:* Jeneen Interlandi, "GRAS: The Hidden Substances in Your Food," *Consumer Reports,* August 17, 2016, https://www.consumerreports.org/food-safety/gras-hidden-ingredients-in -your-food/.

20 *process was minimal:* Ibid.

21 *to be carcinogenic:* T.Y. Liu et. al., "Safrole-induced Oxidative Damage in the Liver of Sprague-Dawley Rats," *Food and Chemical Toxicology* 37, no. 7 (July 1999): 697–702, accessed via Science Direct, https://www.sciencedirect.com/science/article/pii/S0278691599000551?via%3Dihub.

22 *into one sensation:* "How does the way food looks or its smell influence its taste?" *Scientific American,* April 2, 2008, https://www.scientificamerican.com/article/experts-how-does-sight -smell-affect-taste/.

23 *"flavor, not nutrition":* Code of Federal Regulations Title 21.

24 *sugar, and water:* David Andrews, "Synthetic Ingredients in Natural Flavors and Natural Flavors

in Artificial Flavors," Natural vs. Artificial Flavors, Environmental Working Group, accessed November 2020, https://www.ewg.org/foodscores/content/natural-vs-artificial-flavors/.

25   *deemed GRAS:* "Flavor," Natural & Artificial Flavor, Made Safe, accessed November 2020, https://www.madesafe.org/science/hazard-list/flavor/.

26   *hundreds of chemicals:* Gary Reineccius, "What is the Difference between Artificial and Natural Flavors?" *Scientific American,* July 29, 2002, https://www.scientificamerican.com/article/what-is -the-difference-be-2002-07-29/.

27   *directly from nature:* C. Rose Kennedy, "What's in a Flavor," The Flavor Rundown: Natural vs. Artificial Flavors, Harvard University, The Graduate School of Arts and Sciences, September 21, 2015, http://sitn.hms.harvard.edu/flash/2015/the-flavor-rundown-natural-vs-artificial-flavors/.

28   *made from corn:* John S. White, "Straight Talk about High-Fructose Corn Syrup: What It Is and What It Ain't," *The American Journal of Clinical Nutrition* 88, no.6 (December 2008): 1716S-1721S, accessed via Oxford Academic, https://academic.oup.com/ajcn/article/88/6/1716S/4617107.

29   *form of carbohydrates:* "Non-Caloric Sweeteners," UCSF Children's Hospital, based on "Position of the American Dietetic Association: Use of Nutritive and Nonnutritive Sweeteners," *Journal of the American Dietetic Association* 104 (2004): 255–275, https://diabetes.ucsf.edu/sites/diabetes.ucsf .edu/files/PEDS%20Sugar%20and%20Sugar%20Substitutes%20Handout.pdf.

30   *fructose into fat:* Sharon S. Elliott et. al., "Fructose, Weight Gain, and the Insulin Resistance Syndrome," *American Journal of Clinical Nutrition* 76, no.5 (November 2002): 911–22, accessed via PubMed, https://www.ncbi.nlm.nih.gov/pubmed/12399260.

31   *metabolized differently:* M. Akram and Abdul Hamid, "Mini Review on Fructose Metabolism," *Obesity Research & Clinical Practice* 7, no.2 (March/April 2013): e89-e94, accessed via PubMed, https://pubmed.ncbi.nlm.nih.gov/24331770/.

32   *consume in excess:* Ibid.

33   *use it as energy:* Ernst J. Schaefer et. al., "Dietary Fructose and Glucose Differentially Affect Lipid and Glucose Homeostasis," *The Journal of Nutrition* 139, no.6 (June 2009): 1257S-1262S, accessed via U.S. National Library of Medicine, https://www.ncbi.nlm.nih.gov/pmc/articles /PMC2682989/.

34   *contaminated with mercury:* Renee Dufault et. al., "Mercury from Chlor-Alkali Plants: Measured Concentrations in Food Product Sugar," *Environmental Health* 8 (2009), accessed via BMC, https://ehjournal.biomedcentral.com/articles/10.1186/1476-069X-8-2.

35   *31 percent of them:* David Wallinga et. al., "Not So Sweet: Missing Mercury and High Fructose Corn Syrup," Institute for Agriculture and Trade Policy, January 2009, https://www.iatp.org /sites/default/files/421_2_105026.pdf.

36   *also be reported:* Stephen Bose-O'Reilly et. al., "Mercury Exposure and Children's Health," *Current Problems In Pediatric and Adolescent Health Care* 40, no.8 (2010): 186–215, accessed via U.S. National Library of Medicine, https://www.ncbi.nlm.nih.gov/pmc/articles/PMC3096006/.

37   *difficulties years later:* Fulton, Eliza, overview of *Excitotoxins: The Taste That Kills,* by Russell

Blaylock, Clayton College for Natural Health, March 10, 2008, *https://www.infiniteunknown* .net/wp-content/uploads/2011/07/Excitotoxins.pdf.

38 *in the forebrain:* Russell L. Blaylock, *Excitotoxins: The Taste That Kills* (Albuquerque, NM: Health Press, 1997), 12.

39 *cause lesions there:* John R. Brobeck, "Mechanism of the Development of Obesity in Animals with Hypothalamic Lesions," *Physiological Reviews* 26, no.4 (October 1946): 541–559, accessed via American Physiological Society, https://journals.physiology.org/doi/abs/10.1152/phys rev.1946.26.4.541?journalCode=physrev.

40 *tells us we're full:* Ka He et. al., "Association of Monosodium Glutamate Intake with Overweight in Chinese Adults," *Obesity Research Journal* 16, no. 8 (August 2008): 1875–1880, accessed via Wiley Online Library, https://onlinelibrary.wiley.com/doi/full/10.1038/oby.2008.274.

41 *rather the potency:* "All About Glutamate in Food," MSG Facts, accessed November 2020, https:// msgfacts.com/.

42 *MSG within them:* adapted from "Ingredient Names Used to Hide Manufactured free Glutamate (MfG)," Truth in Labeling Campaign, accessed November 2020, https://www.truthinlabeling .org/names.html.

43 *in foods for centuries:* Monica Reinagel, "The Carrageenan Controversy," *Scientific American,* July 1, 2015, https://www.scientificamerican.com/article/the-carrageenan-controversy/.

44 *inflammatory bowel disease:* S. Bhattacharyya et. al., "Exposure to the Common Food Additive Carrageenan Leads to Glucose Intolerance, Insulin Resistance and Inhibition of Insulin Signaling in HepG2 Cells and C57BL/6J Mice," *Diabetologia* 55, no.1 (January 2012): 194–203, accessed via PubMed, https://www.ncbi.nlm.nih.gov/pubmed/22011715.

45 *results aren't conclusive:* Sumit Bhattacharyya et. al., "Distinct Effects of Carrageenan and High-Fat Consumption on the Mechanisms of Insulin Resistance in Nonobese and Obese Models of Type 2 Diabetes," *Journal of Diabetes Research* 2019 (April 2019): 1–14, accessed via Hindawi, https://www.hindawi.com/journals/jdr/2019/9582714/.

46 *to the digestive tracts:* John Vincent Martino et. al., "The Role of Carrageenan and Carboxymthylcellulose in the Development of Intestinal Inflammation," *Frontiers in Pediatrics* 5 (2017): 96, accessed via U.S. National Library of Medicine, https://www.ncbi.nlm.nih.gov/pmc /articles/PMC5410598/.

47 *properties of new drugs:* Sarika Amdekar et. al., "Anti-Inflammatory Activity of Lactobacillus on Carrageenan-Induced Paw Edema in Male Wistar Rats," *International Journal of Inflammation* 2012 (February 2012): 752015, accessed via National Library of Medicine, https://www.ncbi.nlm .nih.gov/pmc/articles/PMC3299308/.

48 *didn't drink diet soda:* Qing Yang, "Gain Weight by 'Going Diet'? Artificial Sweeteners and the Neurobiology of Sugar Cravings," *Yale Journal of Biology and Medicine* 83, no.2 (June 2010): 101–108, accessed via U.S. National Library of Medicine, https://www.ncbi.nlm.nih.gov/pmc /articles/PMC2892765/.

49   *the cephalic response:* Jaapna Dhillon et. al., "The Cephalic Phase Insulin Response to Nutritive and Low-Calorie Sweeteners in Solid and Beverage Form," *Physiology & Behavior* 181 (November 2017): 100–109, accessed via U.S. National Library of Medicine, https://www.ncbi.nlm.nih.gov /pmc/articles/PMC5634742/.

50   *disrupt the gut flora:* "Gut Microbes and Diet Interact to Affect Obesity," National Institutes of Health, September 16, 2013, https://www.nih.gov/news-events/nih-research-matters/gut -microbes-diet-interact-affect-obesity.

51   *hunger and fullness:* Claudia Wallis, "How Gut Bacteria Help Make Us Fat and Thin," *Scientific American,* June 1, 2014, https://www.scientificamerican.com/article/how-gut-bacteria-help -make-us-fat-and-thin/.

52   *rats only, interestingly:* Morando Soffritti et. al., "First Experimental Demonstration of the Multipotential Carcinogenic Effects of Aspartame Administered in the Feed to Sprague-Dawley Rats," *Environmental Health Perspectives* 114, no.3 (March 2006): 379–385, accessed U.S. National Library of Medicine, https://www.ncbi.nlm.nih.gov/pmc/articles/PMC1392232/.

53   *to stay away:* Naveed Saleh, "5 Reasons to Avoid Diet Drinks at All Costs," Food & Diet, MDLinx, December 2, 2019, https://www.mdlinx.com/internal-medicine/article/5280; Sharon E. Jacob and Sarah Stechschulte, "Formaldehyde, Aspartame, and Migraines: A Possible Connections," *Dermatitis* 19, no. 3 (May/June 2008): E10–11, accessed via PubMed, https://pubmed.ncbi.nlm .nih.gov/18627677.

54   *in male mice:* "CSPI Downgrades Sucralose from 'Caution' to 'Avoid'," Center for Science in the Public Interest, February 8, 2016, https://cspinet.org/new/201602081.html.

55   *among other things:* Yu-Jie Zhang et. al., "Impacts of Gut Bacteria on Human Health and Diseases," *International Journal of Molecular Sciences* 16, no. 4 (April 2015): 7493–7519, accessed via U.S. National Library of Medicine, https://www.ncbi.nlm.nih.gov/pmc/articles/PMC44 25030/.

56   *other cancers in mice:* Rajendrakumar M. Patel et. al., "Popular Sweetener Sucralose as a Migraine Trigger," *Headache: The Journal of Head and Face Pain* 46, no.8 (September 2006): 1303–1304, https://headachejournal.onlinelibrary.wiley.com/doi/abs/10.1111/j.1526-4610.2006.00543_1.x; M. Soffriti et. al., "Sucralose Administered in Feed, Beginning Prenatally through Lifespan, Induces Hematopoietic Neoplasias in Male Swiss Mice," *International Journal of Occupational and Environmental Health* 22, no. 1 (January 2016):7–17, accessed via Taylor & Francis Online, https:// www.tandfonline.com/doi/abs/10.1080/10773525.2015.1106075?journalCode=yjoh20.

57   *are potentially toxic:* "Harmful Compounds Might Be Formed When Foods Containing the Sweetener Sucralose Are Heated," BFR Federal Institute for Risk Assessment, via ErekAlert and American Association for the Advancement of Science, April 9, 2019, https://www.eurekalert .org/pub_releases/2019–04/bfif-hcm041219.php.

58   *and cancer in humans:* "Case Study 24: Methylene Chloride Toxicity," in *Environmental Medicine: Integrating a Missing Element into Medical Education,* ed. Laura Welch (Agency for Toxic

Substances and Disease Registry, 1995), accessed via The National Academies Press, https://www.nap.edu/read/4795/chapter/36.

59   *indicated that it is safe:* Myra L. Karstadt, "Testing Needed for Acesulfame Potassium, an Artificial Sweetener," *Environmental Health Perspectives* 114, no. 9 (September 2006): A516, accessed via U.S. National Library of Medicine, https://www.ncbi.nlm.nih.gov/pmc/articles/PMC1570055/.

60   *there is a risk:* M. D. Reuber, "Carcinogenicity of Saccharin," *Environmental Health Perspectives* 25 (August 1978): 173–200, accessed via U.S. National Library of Medicine, https://www.ncbi.nlm.nih.gov/pmc/articles/PMC1637197/.

61   *"a human carcinogen":* "Butylated Hydroxyanisole," from *14th Report on Carcinogens,* U.S. Department of Health and Human Services, 2016, accessed via National Toxicology Program website, https://ntp.niehs.nih.gov/ntp/roc/content/profiles/butylatedhydroxyanisole.pdf.

62   *in mice and rats:* Elizabeth Vavasour, "Butylated Hydroxytoluene (BHT)," Toxicological Evaluation Division, Health Canada, via International Programme on Chemical Safety (IPCS), accessed November 2020, http://www.inchem.org/documents/jecfa/jecmono/v35je02.htm.

63   *hyperactivity in children:* Donna McCann et. al., "Food Additives and Hyperactive Behavior in 3-Year-Old and 8/9-Year-Old Children in the Community: A Randomized, Double-Blinded, Placebo-Controlled Trial," *Lancet* 370, no. 9598 (November 2007): 1560–7, accessed via PubMed, https://pubmed.ncbi.nlm.nih.gov/17825405/.

64   *"experience of school":* Claudia Wallis, "Hyper Kids? Cut Out Preservatives," *TIME,* September 6, 2007, http://content.time.com/time/health/article/0,8599,1659835,00.html.

65   *levels of benzene:* "Questions and Answers on the Occurrence of Benzene in Soft Drinks and Other Beverages," U.S. Food & Drug Administration, last updated January 24, 2018, https://www.fda.gov/food/chemicals/questions-and-answers-occurrence-benzene-soft-drinks-and-other-beverages; Vania Paula Salviano Dos Santos et. al., "Benzene as a Chemical Hazard in Processed Foods," *International Journal of Food Science* 2015 (2015): 545640, accessed via PubMed, https://www.ncbi.nlm.nih.gov/pubmed/26904662.

66   *"lymphocytes in vitro":* N. Zengin et. al., "The Evaluation of the Genotoxicity of Two Food Preservatives: Sodium Benzoate and Potassium Benzoate," *Food and Chemical Toxicology* 49, no. 4 (April 2011): 763–9, accessed via PubMed, https://pubmed.ncbi.nlm.nih.gov/21130826/.

67   *in humans and animals:* Carol Potera, "Diet and Nutrition: The Artificial Food Dye Blues," *Environmental Health Perspectives* 118, no. 10 (October 2010): A428, accessed via U.S. National Library of Medicine, https://www.ncbi.nlm.nih.gov/pmc/articles/PMC2957945/.

68   *swelling and flushing:* "Food Coloring Allergy," New York Allergy & Sinus Centers, accessed November 2020, https://www.nyallergy.com/food-coloring-allergy.

69   *reported with carmine:* B. Wuthrich et. al., "Anaphylactic Reaction to Ingested Carmine (E120)," *Allergy* 52, no. 11 (November 1997): 1133–7, accessed via PubMed, https://pubmed.ncbi.nlm.nih.gov/9404569/.

70   *"they have ADHD":* L. Eugene Arnold et. al., "Artificial Food Colors and Attention-Deficit /Hyperactivity Symptoms: Conclusions to Dye For," *Neurotherapeutics* 9, no. 3 (July 2012): 599– 609, accessed via PubMed, https://pubmed.ncbi.nlm.nih.gov/22864801/.

71   *"attention in children":* "Food additives," U.K. Food Standards Agency, last updated October 14, 2019, https://www.food.gov.uk/safety-hygiene/food-additives.

72   *and corn plants:* "The Basics: Start Here," Institute for Responsible Technology, accessed November 2020, https://www.responsibletechnology.org/the-basics/.

73   *only a few days:* Megan L. Norris, "Will GMOs Hurt My Body?," Harvard University, The Graduate School of Arts and Sciences, August 10, 2015, http://sitn.hms.harvard.edu/flash/2015 /will-gmos-hurt-my-body/.

74   *"an ongoing battle":* Ibid.

Chapter 6. Safe Water, Food Storage, and the Kitchen Cleanout

1   *hard, clear plastic:* Brent A. Bauer, "What is BPA, and What Are the Concerns about BPA?" Nutrition and Healthy Eating, Mayo Clinic, December 18, 2019, https://www.mayoclinic.org /healthy-lifestyle/nutrition-and-healthy-eating/expert-answers/bpa/faq-20058331.

2   *and even infertility:* Chris E. Talsness, "Components of Plastic: Experimental Studies in Animals and Relevance for Human Health," *Philosophical Transactions, Series B: Biological Sciences* 364, no. 1526 (2009): 2079–96, accessed via U.S. National Library of Medicine, https://www.ncbi.nlm .nih.gov/pmc/articles/PMC2873015/.

3   *to learning disabilities:* "Chemical Present in Clear Plastics Can Impair Learning and Cause Disease," Yale News, March 28, 2005, https://news.yale.edu/2005/03/28/chemical-present-clear -plastics-can-impair-learning-and-cause-disease.

4   *are produced each year:* "Q&A: Bisphenol A and Plastics," Johns Hopkins Bloomberg School of Public Health, June 23, 2008, https://www.jhsph.edu/news/stories/2008/goldman-schwab-bpa.html.

5   *hands were dry:* Annette M. Hormann et. al., "Holding Thermal Receipt Paper and Eating Food after Using Hand Sanitizer Results in High Serum Bioactive and Urine Total Levels of Bispheno A (BPA)," *PLOS ONE* 9, no. 10 (2014): e110509, accessed via U.S. National Library of Medicine, https://www.ncbi.nlm.nih.gov/pmc/articles/PMC4206219/?fbclid=IwAR3xfJcFmUUIyb6a1ze -_uZC4JAANCYKUEL3J1x4dv6bCIno635cEEgyYAQ.

6   *and cardiovascular systems:* Alberto Leonardi et. al., "The Effect of Bisphenol A on Puberty: A Critical Review of the Medical Literature," *International Journal of Environmental Research and Public Health* 14, no. 9 (September 2017): 1044, accessed via U.S. National Library of Medicine, https://www.ncbi.nlm.nih.gov/pmc/articles/PMC5615581/.

7   *behavior issues in children:* Frederica Perera et. al., "Bisphenol A Exposure and Symptoms of Anxiety and Depression Among Inner City Children at 10–12 Years of Age," *Environmental Research* 151 (November 2016): 195–202, accessed via U.S. National Library of Medicine, https:// www.ncbi.nlm.nih.gov/pmc/articles/PMC5071142/.

8   *neurodevelopmental issues:* "More Evidence That BPA Found in Clear Plastics Impairs Brain Function," Yale News, September 3, 2008, https://news.yale.edu/2008/09/03/more-evidence -bpa-found-clear-plastics-impairs-brain-function.

9   *disruptive heart rhythms:* Endocrine Society, "Common BPA-like Chemical, BPS, Disrupts Heart Rhythms in Females," *News Wise,* June 23, 2014, https://www.newswise.com/articles/common -bpa-like-chemical-bps-disrupts-heart-rhythms-in-females.

10   *BPS and weight gain:* Melanie H. Jacobson et. al., "Urinary Bisphenols and Obesity Prevalence Among U.S. Children and Adolescents," *Journal of the Endocrine Society* 3, not. 9 (September 2019), 1715–1726, accessed via Oxford Academic, https://academic.oup.com/jes/article/3/9/1715/5537531.

11   *brain development and behavior:* Mary C. Catanese et. al., "Bisphenol S (BPS) Alters Maternal Behavior and Brain in Mice Exposed During Pregnancy/Lactation and Their Daughters," *Endocrinology* 158, no. 3 (March 2017): 516–530, accessed via Oxford Academic, https://academic .oup.com/endo/article/158/3/516/3053388.

12   *in the hypothalamus:* Cassandra D. Kinch et. al., "Low-Dose Exposure to Bisphenol a and Replacement Bisphenol S Induces Precocious Hypothalamic Neurogenesis in Embryonic Zebrafish," *Proceedings of the National Academy of Sciences of the USA* 112, no. 5 (February 2015): 1475–1480, accessed via U.S. National Library of Medicine, https://www.ncbi.nlm.nih.gov/pmc /articles/PMC4321238/.

13   *$1.47 billion:* Jan Conway, "Retail Sales of Non-Stick Cookware in the U.S. 2010–2019," Furniture, Furnishings & Household Items, *Statista,* March 2, 2020, https://www.statista.com /statistics/515115/us-retail-sales-of-non-stick-cookware/.

14   *and nonreactive surface:* Daisy Coyle, "Is Nonstick Cookware Like Teflon Safe to Use?" *Healthline,* July 13, 2017, https://www.healthline.com/nutrition/nonstick-cookware-safety.

15   *illnesses each year:* "Canaries in the Kitchen: Teflon Toxicosis," Environmental Working Group, May 15, 2003, https://www.ewg.org/research/canaries-kitchen.

16   *other neurodegenerative diseases:* Layla A. Al Juhaiman, "Estimating Aluminum Leaching from Aluminum Cook Wares in Different Meat Extracts and Milk," *Journal of Saudi Chemical Society* 14, no. 1 (January 2010): 131–137, accessed via Science Direct, https://www.sciencedirect .com/science/article/pii/S1319610309000751; Jeffery D. Weidenhamer, "Metal Exposures from Aluminum Cookware: An Unrecognized Public Health Risk in Developing Countries," *Science of the Total Environment* 579, no. 1 (February 2017): 805–813, accessed via Science Direct, https:// www.sciencedirect.com/science/article/pii/S0048969716324548.

17   *it's not recommended:* Kristine Lewis, "Products, Brands, and Other Recommendations to Bring the Cookbook to Life," Cooking for Hemochromatosis Resources, Hemochromatosis Help, https://hemochromatosishelp.com/resources/.

18   *"in non-iron utensils":* H.C. Brittin and C. E. Nossaman, "Iron Content of Food Cooked in Iron Utensils," *Journal of the American Diet Association* 86, no. 7 (1986): 897–901, accessed via PubMed, https://pubmed.ncbi.nlm.nih.gov/3722654/.

19   *reseasoning the cookware:* "How to Clean Cast Iron Cookware," Lodge Cast Iron, accessed November 2020, https://www.lodgecastiron.com/discover/cleaning-and-care/cast-iron/how-clean-cast-iron.

20   *in its composition:* Kristin L. Kamerud et. al., "Stainless Steel Leaches Nickel and Chromium into Foods During Cooking," *Journal of Agriculture and Food Chemistry* 61, no. 39 (2013): 9495–501, accessed via U.S. National Library of Medicine, https://www.ncbi.nlm.nih.gov/pmc/articles/PMC4284091/.

21   *have a nickel sensitivity:* "Stainless Steel: The Role of Nickel," Nickel Institute, accessed November 2020, https://nickelinstitute.org/about-nickel/stainless-steel.

22   *60 percent of water:* "The Water in You: Water and the Human Body," Water Science School, U.S. Geological Survey, accessed November 2020, https://www.usgs.gov/special-topic/water-science-school/science/water-you-water-and-human-body?qt-science_center_objects=0#qt-science_center_objects.

23   *forty-five million people:* Maura Allaire, et. al., "National Trends in Drinking Water Quality Violations," *Proceeding of the National Academy of Sciences of the U.S.A.* 115, no. 9 (February 2018): 2078–2083, accessed via U.S. National Library of Medicine, https://www.ncbi.nlm.nih.gov/pmc/articles/PMC5834717/.

24   *comparable to bottled water:* Katherine Zeratsky, "Is Tap Water as Safe as Bottled Water?" Nutrition and Healthy Eating, Mayo Clinic, March 19, 2020, https://www.mayoclinic.org/healthy-lifestyle/nutrition-and-healthy-eating/expert-answers/tap-vs-bottled-water/faq-20058017.

25   *can be contaminated:* Ryan Felton, "Should We Break Our Bottled Water Habit?" *Consumer Reports,* October 9, 2019, https://www.consumerreports.org/bottled-water/should-we-break-our-bottled-water-habit/.

26   *the water you drink:* EWG's Tap Water Database: 2019 Update, Environmental Working Group, accessed November 2020, https://www.ewg.org/tapwater/.

27   *qualities of your water:* "Step-by-Step Guide to Selecting a Home Tap Water Filter," EWG's Tap Water Database: 2019 Update, Environmental Working Group, accessed November 2020, https://www.ewg.org/tapwater/water-filter-step-by-step-guide.php.

28   *comes from the tap:* "Take Back the Tap: The Big Business Hustle of Bottled Water," Food & Water Watch, February 2018, https://www.foodandwaterwatch.org/sites/default/files/rpt_1802_tbttbigwaterhustle-web.pdf.

29   *"sometimes not":* Andrew Postman, "The Truth About Tap," Natural Resources Defense Council, January 5, 2016, https://www.nrdc.org/stories/truth-about-tap.

30   *extended period of time:* Ryan Felton, "Arsenic in Some Bottled Water Brands at Unsafe Levels, Consumer Reports Says," *Consumer Reports,* June 28, 2019, https://www.consumerreports.org/water-quality/arsenic-in-some-bottled-water-brands-at-unsafe-levels/.

31   *like cardiovascular disease:* "Arsenic," Fact Sheets, World Health Organization, February 15, 2018, https://www.who.int/news-room/fact-sheets/detail/arsenic.

32   *little as ten weeks:* Leonard Sax, "Polyethylene Terephthalate May Yield Endocrine Disruptors,"
     Environmental Health Perspectives 118, no. 4 (April 2010): 445–448, accessed via U.S. National
     Library of Medicine, https://www.ncbi.nlm.nih.gov/pmc/articles/PMC2854718/.

33   *since the 1950s:* Matthew Taylor, "Plastic Pollution Risks 'near Permanent Contamination of
     Natural Environment,'" *The Guardian,* July 19, 2017, https://www.theguardian.com/environment
     /2017/jul/19/plastic-pollution-risks-near-permanent-contamination-of-natural-environment.

34   *purchased every minute:* Sandra Laville and Matthew Taylor, "A Million Bottles a Minute: World's
     Plastic Binge 'as Dangerous as Climate Change'," *The Guardian,* June 28, 2017, https://www
     .theguardian.com/environment/2017/jun/28/a-million-a-minute-worlds-plastic-bottle-binge
     -as-dangerous-as-climate-change.

35   *more than tap:* Matthew Boesler, "Bottled Water Costs 2000 Times As Much As Tap Water,"
     Business Insider, July 12, 2013, https://www.businessinsider.com/bottled-water-costs-2000x
     -more-than-tap-2013–7.

36   *in everyday plastics:* Lisa Zimmermann et. al., "Benchmarking the in Vitro Toxicity and Chemical
     Composition of Plastic Consumer Products," *Environmental Science & Technology* 53, no. 19 (2019):
     11467–11477, accessed via ACS Publications, https://pubs.acs.org/doi/abs/10.1021/acs.est.9b02293.

Chapter 7. Don't Be Fooled by Cosmetic Labels

1   *"astoundingly limited":* Editorial Board, "Do You Know What's in Your Cosmetics?" *The New
    York Times,* September 2, 2019, https://www.nytimes.com/2019/02/09/opinion/cosmetics-safety
    -makeup.html.

2   *"go on the market":* "FDA Authority Over Cosmetics: How Cosmetics Are Not FDA-Approved,
    but Are FDA-Regulated," U.S. Food & Drug Administration, last updated August 24, 2020,
    https://www.fda.gov/cosmetics/cosmetics-laws-regulations/fda-authority-over-cosmetics-how
    -cosmetics-are-not-fda-approved-are-fda-regulated.

3   *personal care products:* "EWG's Skin Deep," Environmental Working Group, accessed November
    2020, https://www.ewg.org/skindeep/contents/about-page/.

4   *and Unilever:* "Celebrating 125 Years of Achievement: Year in Review 2019," Personal Care
    Products Council, December 2019, https://www.personalcarecouncil.org/wp-content/up
    loads/2020/02/PCPC_YIR2019.pdf.

5   *banned just eleven:* "International Laws," Campaign for Safe Cosmetics, July 2013, http://www
    .safecosmetics.org/get-the-facts/regulations/international-laws/.

6   *penetration enhancers:* "About EWG's Skin Deep," Environmental Working Group, accessed
    November 2020, https://www.ewg.org/skindeep/contents/about-page/.

7   *since 1938!:* Scott Faber, "80 Years Later, Cosmetics Chemicals Still Unregulated," Environmental
    Working Group, June 25, 2018, https://www.ewg.org/news-and-analysis/2018/06/80-years-later
    -cosmetics-chemicals-still-unregulated.

8   *than adults are:* Technical Panel, "Supplemental Guidance for Assessing Susceptibility from

Early-Life Exposure to Carcinogens," Risk Assessment Forum, U.S. Environmental Protection Agency, March 2005, https://www.epa.gov/sites/production/files/2013–09/documents/childrens _supplement_final.pdf.

9   *immune system disfunction:* "Exposure to Multiple Chemicals in Consumer Products During Early Pregnancy Is Related to Lower IQ in Children," Mount Sinai, October 24, 2019, https:// www.mountsinai.org/about/newsroom/2019/exposure-to-multiple-chemicals-in-consumer -products-during-early-pregnancy-is-related-to-lower-iq-in-children; "Mount Sinai Children's Environmental Health Center Publishes a List of the Top Ten Toxic Chemicals Suspected to Cause Autism and Learning Disabilities," Mount Sinai, April 25, 2012, https://www.mountsinai .org/about/newsroom/2012/mount-sinai-childrens-environmental-health-center-publishes -a-list-of-the-top-ten-toxic-chemicals-suspected-to-cause-autism-and-learning-disabilities; "Exposure to Three Classes of Common Chemicals May Affects Female Development," Mount Sinai, April 5, 2010, https://www.mountsinai.org/about/newsroom/2010/exposure -to-three-classes-of-common-chemicals-may-affect-female-development; "Mount Sinai Led Study Finds Prenatal Exposure to Certain Manmade Chemicals Negatively Affects Childhood Neurodevelopment," Mount Sinai, January 26, 2010, https://www.mountsinai.org/about /newsroom/2010/mount-sinailed-study-finds-prenatal-exposure-to-certain-manmade-chemicals -negatively-affects-childhood-neurodevelopment.

10   *in human history:* Tara Parker-Pope, "Obesity Rates Stall, But Not Decline," *The New York Times,* January 17, 2012, https://well.blogs.nytimes.com/2012/01/17/obesity-rates-stall-but-no-decline/.

11   *at age seven:* "How Girls Are Developing Earlier in an Age of 'New Puberty'," *Fresh Air,* December 2, 2014, https://www.npr.org/sections/health-shots/2014/12/02/367811777/how-girls-are-developing -earlier-in-an-age-of-new-puberty.

12   *earlier now too:* "Like Girls, Boys Are Entering Puberty Earlier," *Morning Edition,* December 24, 2012, https://www.npr.org/sections/health-shots/2012/12/24/167735056/like-girls-boys-are -entering-puberty-earlier.

13   *entering puberty earlier:* Sheena Scruggs, "Earlier Puberty Linked with Personal Care Products," *Environmental Factor,* January 2019, https://factor.niehs.nih.gov/2019/1/papers/puberty/index.htm.

14   *and emotional health:* "Teen Girls' Body Burden of Hormone-Altering Cosmetics Chemicals," Environmental Working Group, September 24, 2008, https://www.ewg.org/research/teen-girls -body-burden-hormone-altering-cosmetics-chemicals/teens-are-vulnerable.

15   *growth of bacteria:* Brenda Goodman, "FAQ: Parabens and Breast Cancer," *WebMD,* October 27, 2015, https://www.webmd.com/breast-cancer/news/20151027/parabens-breast-cancer#1.

16   *and bioaccumulation:* "Red List," Campaign for Safe Cosmetics, accessed November 2020, http:// www.safecosmetics.org/take-action/businesses-and-retailers/red-list/.

17   *on advertising:* A. Guttmann, "U.S. Perfumes, Cosmetics, and Other Toilet Preparations Ad Spend 2018–2019," *Statista,* November 5, 2020, https://www.statista.com/statistics/470467 /perfumes-cosmetics-and-other-toilet-preparations-industry-ad-spend-usa/.

18   *of personal care products:* "Fact Sheet: Potentially Toxic Chemicals in Personal Care Products," NYS Health Foundation, June 4, 2018, http://www.ny2aap.org/pdf/Potentially ToxicChemicalsPersonalCareProducts.pdf.

19   *products each day:* Statista Research Department, "Frequency of makeup use among U.S. consumers 2017, by age," *Statista,* December 20, 2019, https://www.statista.com/statistics/713178 /makeup-use-frequency-by-age/.

20   *168 chemical ingredients:* Sydney Lupkin, "Women Put an Average of 168 Chemicals on Their Bodies Each Day, Consumer Group Says," *ABC News,* April 27, 2015, https://abcnews.go.com /Health/women-put-average-168-chemicals-bodies-day-consumer/story?id=30615324 .

21   *their body each year:* Paul Stokes, "Body Absorbs 5lbs of Make Up Chemicals a Year," *The Telegraph,* June 21, 2007, https://www.telegraph.co.uk/news/uknews/1555173/Body-absorbs-5lb -of-make-up-chemicals-a-year.html.

22   *and temperature control:* "Skin Exposures & Effects," Centers for Disease Control and Prevention, last reviewed July 2, 2013, based on National Institute for Occupational Safety and Health, https://www.cdc.gov/niosh/topics/skin/.

23   *prolonging exposure:* American Chemical Society, "Triclosan Accumulates in Toothbrushes, Potentially Prolonging Users' Exposure," *ScienceDaily,* October 25, 2017, https://www .sciencedaily.com/releases/2017/10/171025090454.htm.

24   *of human breast milk:* Lisa M. Weatherly and Julie A. Gosse, "Triclosan Exposure, Transformation, and Human Health Effects," *Journal of Toxicology and Environmental Health* 20, no. 8 (2017): 447–469, accessed via U.S. National Library of Medicine, https://www.ncbi.nlm.nih.gov/pmc /articles/PMC6126357/.

25   *to antibiotic-resistant "superbugs":* Ji Lu et. al., "Non-Antibiotic Antimicrobial Triclosan Induces Multiple Antibiotic Resistance through Genetic Mutation," *Environmental International* 118, (September 2018): 257–265, accessed via Science Direct, https://www.sciencedirect.com/science /article/pii/S0160412018303672?via%3Dihub.

26   *a normal household:* "Antibacterial Soap? You Can Skip It, Use Plain Soap and Water," U.S. Food & Drug Administration, last updated May 16, 2019, https://www.fda.gov/consumers/consumer -updates/antibacterial-soap-you-can-skip-it-use-plain-soap-and-water.

27   *EPA's allowable amount:* E. Matthew Fiss et. al., "Formation of Chloroform and Other Chlorinated Byproducts by Chlorination of Triclosan-Containing Antibacterial Products," *Environmental Science & Technology* 41, not. 7 (2007): 2387–2394, accessed via ACA Publications, https://pubs .acs.org/doi/10.1021/es062227l.

28   *"plain soap and water":* "Antibacterial Soap? You Can Skip It, Use Plain Soap and Water," U.S. Food & Drug Administration.

29   *decision-making process:* Babu John Mariadoss, "Factors That Influence Consumers' Buying Behavior," *Core Principles of Marketing,* 2017, accessed via Press Books, https://opentext.wsu.edu /marketing/chapter/5-1-factors-that-influence-consumers-buying-behavior/.

30   *$31 billion by 2026:* "Flavors & Fragrances Market To Reach USD 31.38 Billion By 2026," *Reports and Data,* September 18, 2019, https://www.globenewswire.com/news-release/2019/09/18/1917609 /0/en/Flavors-Fragrances-Market-To-Reach-USD-31-38-Billion-By-2026-Reports-And-Data .html.

31   *four major companies:* David Andrews, "Synthetic ingredients in Natural Flavors and Natural Flavors in Artificial flavors," Environmental Working Group, accessed November 2020, https:// www.ewg.org/foodscores/content/natural-vs-artificial-flavors/.

32   *popcorn is designed:* C. Rose Kennedy, "What's in a Flavor," Harvard University, The Graduate School of Arts and Sciences, September 21, 2015, http://sitn.hms.harvard.edu/flash/2015/the -flavor-rundown-natural-vs-artificial-flavors/.

33   *a fragrance formulation:* "IFRA Transparency List," International Fragrance Association, accessed November 2020, https://ifrafragrance.org/initiatives/transparency/ifra-transparency-list.

34   *top five allergens:* "Review ACDS' Allergen of the Year 2000–2015," *Dermatologist* 22, no. 11 (November 2014), https://www.the-dermatologist.com/content/review-acds'-allergen-od-year -2000-2015.

35   *and respiratory system:* "Technical Fact Sheet—1.4-Dioxane," U.S. Environmental Protection Agency, November 2017, https://www.epa.gov/sites/production/files/2014-03/documents/ffrro _factsheet_contaminant_14-dioxane_january2014_final.pdf.

36   *the mouth area:* Scientific Committee on Consumer Safety, "Opinion on Phenoxyethanol," European Commission, October 6, 2016, https://ec.europa.eu/health/scientific_committees /consumer_safety/docs/sccs_o_195.pdf.

37   *"and diarrhea":* "U.S. FDA Warns Consumers Against Using Mommy's Bliss Nipple Cream," Saudi Food & Drug Authority, June 1, 2008, https://www.sfda.gov.sa/en/drug/news/pages/332 -ar-01-6.aspx.

38   *and nervous system:* "Is Phenoxyethanol Safe?" *The Derm Review,* August 27, 2020, https:// thedermreview.com/phenoxyethanol/.

39   *via oral exposure:* "Phenol: Hazard Summary 108-95-2," U.S. Environmental Protection Agency, updated January 2000, https://www.epa.gov/sites/production/files/2016-09/documents/phenol.pdf.

40   *and Philip Landrigan:* P. Grandjean and P.J. Landrigan, "Developmental neurotoxicity of industrial chemicals," thelancet.com, published online November 8, 2006, https://www.env -health.org/IMG/pdf/06tl9094page.pdf.

41   *and vertigo:* "Phenol Acute Exposure Guideline Levels," in *Acute Exposure Guideline Levels for Selected Airborne Chemicals: Volume 7,* National Academy of Sciences, 2009, accessed via U.S. National Library of Medicine, https://www.ncbi.nlm.nih.gov/books/NBK214904/.

42   *known to cause cancer:* W.T. Stott et. el., "Evaluation of the Potential of Triethanolamine to Alter Hepatic Choline Levels in Female B6C3F1," *Toxicological Sciences* 79, no. 2 (2004): 242–7, accessed via U.S. National Library of Medicine, https://www.ncbi.nlm.nih.gov/pmc/articles /PMC1592523/; "N-Nitrosamines: 15 Listings," from *14th Report on Carcinogens,* U.S. Department

of Health and Human Services, 2016, accessed via National Toxicology Program website, https://ntp.niehs.nih.gov/ntp/roc/content/profiles/nitrosamines.pdf.

43 *from crude oil:* Birgit Geueke, "Mineral Oil Hydrocarbons," *Food Packaging Forum*, June 30, 2017, https://www.foodpackagingforum.org/food-packaging-health/mineral-oil-hydrocarbons#:~:

44 *in the human body:* Nicole Concin et. al., "Evidence for Cosmetics as a Source of Mineral Oil Contamination in Women," *Journal of Women's Health* 20, no. 11 (November 2011): 1713–9, accessed via PubMed, https://www.ncbi.nlm.nih.gov/pubmed/21970597.

45 *as in food packaging:* Ralph Pirow et. al., "Mineral Oil in Food, Cosmetic Products, and in Products Regulated by Other Legislations," *Critical Reviews in Toxicology* 49, no. 9 (October 2019): 742–789, accessed via PubMed, https://pubmed.ncbi.nlm.nih.gov/31939687/.

46 *causes health risks:* "Mineral Oil Hydrocarbons: EFSA Publishes Opinion on These Complex Compounds," European Food and Safety Authority, June 6, 2012, https://www.efsa.europa.eu/en/press/news/120606.

47 *sources, including cosmetics:* Wiley-Blackwell, "Mineral Oil Contamination in Humans: A Health Problem?" *ScienceDaily,* November 24, 2008, https://www.sciencedaily.com/releases/2008/11/081124102706.htm.

48 *or palm kernel oil:* "Sodium Lauryl Sulfate," ChemicalSafetyFacts.org, accessed November 2020, https://www.chemicalsafetyfacts.org/sodium-lauryl-sulfate/.

49 *an known human carcinogen:* Britt E. Erickson, "EPA Deems Ethylene Oxide A Carcinogen," *Chemical & Engineering News* vol. 92, no. 34, August 25, 2014, https://cen.acs.org/articles/92/i34/EPA-Deems-Ethylene-Oxide-Carcinogen.html.

50 *to heal the skin:* Tove Agner and Jorgen Serup, "Sodium Lauryl Sulphate for Irritant Patch Testing—A Dose-Response Study Using Bioengineering Methods for Determination of Skin Irritation," *Journal of Investigative Dermatology* 95, no. 5 (November 1990): 543–547, accessed via Science Direct, https://www.sciencedirect.com/science/article/pii/S0022202X9091287L.

51 *vulnerable to irritants:* B.B. Herlofson and P. Barkvoll, "Sodium Lauryl Sulfate and Recurrent Aphthous Ulcers. A Preliminary Study," *Acta Odontologica Scandinavica* 52, no. 5 (October 1994): 257–9, accessed via PubMed, https://www.ncbi.nlm.nih.gov/pubmed/7825393.

52 *probable human carcinogen:* "Technical Fact Sheet—1,4 Dioxane," U.S. Environmental Protection Agency, November 2017, https://www.epa.gov/sites/production/files/2014-03/documents/ffrro_factsheet_contaminant_14-dioxane_january2014_final.pdf.

53 *residue can remain:* "DRS Dioxane Removal System," Chemithon Corporation, 2013, http://www.chemithon.com/Proc_drs.html.

54 *to be a neurotoxin:* Kai He et. al., "Methylisothiazolinone, a Neurotoxic Biocide, Disrupts the Association of Src Family Tyrosine Kinases with Focal Adhesion Kinase in Developing Cortical Neurons," *The Journal of Pharmacology and Experimental Therapeutics* 317, no. 3 (June 2006): 1320–9, accessed via PubMed, https://www.ncbi.nlm.nih.gov/pubmed/16547166.

55 *conditions, and cancer:* Megan J. Schlichte and Rajani Katta, "Methylisothiazolinone: An

Emergent Allergen in Common Pediatric Skin Care Products," *Dermatology Research and Practice* 2014 (2014): 132564, accessed via U.S. National Library of Medicine, https://www.ncbi.nlm.nih .gov/pmc/articles/PMC4197884/.

56   *toxic to human skin:* "Methylisothiazolinone," EWG's Skin Deep, Environmental Working Group, accessed November 2020, https://www.ewg.org/skindeep/ingredients/703935-methy lisothiazolinone/.

57   *negative clinical effects:* Mari Paz Castanedo-Tardana and Kathryn A. Zug, "Methylisothiazolinone," *Dermatisis* 24, no.1 (Jan/Feb 2013): 2–6, accessed via PubMed, https://www.ncbi.nlm.nih.gov /pubmed/23340392.

58   *disabilities, and autism:* University of Pittsburgh Medical Center, "Before Using That Shampoo, Read the Label: Pitt Study Finds Common Ingredient Affects Developing Neurons of Rats," *ScienceDaily,* December 9, 2004, https://www.sciencedaily.com/releases/2004/12/041206204555 .htm.

59   *these types of products:* Scientific Committee on Consumer Safety, "Opinion of Methylisothiazolinone (MI) (P94) Submission III (Sensitisation only)," European Commission, June 25, 2015, https://ec.europa.eu/health/scientific_committees/consumer_safety/docs/sccs _o_178.pdf.

Chapter 8. Change Your Body Wash and Lose Weight

1   *connected to obesity:* Jerrold J. Heindel, "History of the Obesogen Field: Looking Back to Look Forward," *Frontiers in Endocrinology,* January 29, 2019, https://www.frontiersin.org /articles/10.3389/fendo.2019.00014/full.

2   *exposure to toxins:* Caroline H.D. Fall and Kalyanaraman Kumaran, "Metabolic Programming in Early Life in Humans," *Philosophical Transactions Series B: Biological Sciences* 374, no. 1770 (2019): 20180123, accessed via U.S. National Library of Medicine, https://www.ncbi.nlm.nih.gov/pmc /articles/PMC6460078/.

3   *and type 2 diabetes:* Mayo Clinic Staff, "Metabolic syndrome," Mayo Clinic, accessed November 2020, https://www.mayoclinic.org/diseases-conditions/metabolic-syndrome/symptoms-causes /syc-20351916.

4   *want, of course!:* "Obesogen," Science Direct, accessed November 2020, https://www.sciencedirect .com/topics/neuroscience/obesogen.

5   *first year of life:* Claire Philippat et. al., "Prenatal Exposure to Phenols and Growth in Boys," *Epidemiology* 25, no.5 (September 2014): 625–635, accessed via Ovid, https://insights.ovid.com /article/00001648-201409000-00003.

6   *later in childhood:* "Prenatal and Early Life Influences," Obesity Prevention Source, Harvard T. H. Chan School of Public Health, accessed November 2020, https://www.hsph.harvard.edu /obesity-prevention-source/obesity-causes/prenatal-postnatal-obesity/.

7   *breast cancer tumors:* P.D. Darbre et. al., "Concentrations of Parabens in Human Breast Tumours,"

Journal of Applied Toxicology 24, no.1 (Jan/Feb 2004): 5–13, accessed via Pub Med, https://www.ncbi.nlm.nih.gov/pubmed/14745841.

8 *to mimic estrogen:* Wei Yue et. al., "Effects of Estrogen on Breast Cancer Development: Role of Estrogen Receptor Independent Mechanisms," *International Journal of Cancer* 127, no. 8 (October 2010): 1748–1757, accessed via U.S. National Library of Medicine, https://www.ncbi.nlm.nih.gov/pmc/articles/PMC4775086/.

9 *hormone-receptor-positive breast cancers:* "Exposure to Chemicals in Cosmetics," BreastCancer.org, last updated September 11, 2020, https://www.breastcancer.org/risk/factors/cosmetics#:~:text=Parabens%20can%20penetrate%20the%20skin,%2Dreceptor%2Dpositive%20breast%20cancers.

10 *even in tiny amounts:* Shawn Pan et. al., "Parabens and Human Epidermal Growth Factor Receptor Ligand Cross-Talk in Breast Cancer Cells," *Environmental Health Perspectives* 124, no. 5 (May 2016): 563–569, https://ehp.niehs.nih.gov/doi/10.1289/ehp.1409200.

11 *body pretty quickly:* "Parabens Fact Sheet," National Biomonitoring Program, Centers for Disease Control and Prevention, last updated April 7,2017, https://www.cdc.gov/biomonitoring/Parabens_FactSheet.html.

12 *exposure to triclosan:* Michael T. Dinwiddle et. al., "Recent Evidence Regarding Triclosan and Cancer Risk," *International Journal of Environmental Research and Public Health* 11, no. 2 (February 2014): 2209–2217, accessed U.S. National Library of Medicine, https://www.ncbi.nlm.nih.gov/pmc/articles/PMC3945593/.

13 *probable human carcinogen:* "Di(2-ethylhexyl) Phthalate CAS No. 117-81-7," from *14th Report on Carcinogens,* U.S. Department of Health and Human Services, 2016, accessed via National Toxicology Program website, https://ntp.niehs.nih.gov/ntp/roc/content/profiles/diethylhexylphthalate.pdf.

14 *had prenatal exposure:* Pam Factor-Litvak et. al., "Persistent Association between Maternal Prenatal Exposure to Phthalates on Child IQ at Age 7 Years," *PLOS One* 9, no. 12 (December 2014): e114003, accessed via National Library of Medicine, https://www.ncbi.nlm.nih.gov/pmc/articles/PMC4262205/.

15 *in a similar study:* Malene Boas et. al., "Childhood Exposure to Phthalates: Associations with Thyroid Function, Insulin-like Growth Factor I, and Growth," *Environmental Health Perspectives* 118, no. 10 (October 2010): 1458–1464, accessed via U.S. National Library of Medicine, https://www.ncbi.nlm.nih.gov/pmc/articles/PMC2957929/.

16 *cancer. and diabetes:* Katherine Zeratsky, "What Are the Risks of Vitamin D Deficiency?" Nutrition and Healthy Eating, Mayo Clinic, August 27, 2020, https://www.mayoclinic.org/healthy-lifestyle/nutrition-and-healthy-eating/expert-answers/vitamin-d-deficiency/faq-20058397.

17 *levels sufficiently high:* "Radiation: The Known Health Effects of Ultraviolet Radiation," World Health Organization, October 16, 2017, https://www.who.int/news-room/q-a-detail/the-known-health-effects-of-uv.

18   *of developing melanoma:* David G. Hoel et. al., "The Risks and Benefits of Sun Exposure 2016,"
     Dermato-Endocrinology 8, no. 1 (Jan/Dec 2016): e1248325, accessed via U.S. National Library of
     Medicine, https://www.ncbi.nlm.nih.gov/pmc/articles/PMC5129901/.

19   *high during midday:* Prakesh Chandra et. al., "Treatment of Vitamin D Deficiency with UV Light
     in Patients with Malabsorption Syndromes: A Case Series," *Photodermatology Photoimmunology*
     & Photomedicine 23, no. 5 (2007): 179–185, accessed via U.S. National Library of Medicine,
     accessed via U.S. National Library of Medicine, https://www.ncbi.nlm.nih.gov/pmc/articles
     /PMC2846322/; Asta Juzeniene and Johan Moan, "Beneficial Effects of UV Radiation Other than
     via Vitamin D Production," *Dermato-Endocrinology* 4, no. 2 (April 2012): 109–117, accessed via
     U.S. National Library of Medicine, https://www.ncbi.nlm.nih.gov/pmc/articles/PMC3427189/.

20   *in increased toxicity:* Hannah V. Stein et. al., "Photolysis and Cellular Toxicities of the Organic
     Ultraviolet Filter Chemical Octyl Methoxycinnamate and Its Photoproducts," *Environmental*
     Science: Processes & Impacts 19, no. 6 (June 2017): 851–860, accessed via PubMed, https://pubmed
     .ncbi.nlm.nih.gov/28534578/.

21   *and brain signaling:* "Octinoxate," Campaign for Safe Cosmetics, accessed November 2020,
     http://www.safecosmetics.org/get-the-facts/chemicals-of-concern/octinoxate/.

22   *some hormones work:* Stacy Simon, "How Safe is Your Sunscreen?" American Cancer Society,
     August 9, 2018, https://www.cancer.org/latest-news/how-safe-is-your-sunscreen.html.

23   *(turf and lawns):* "Homosalate," EWG's Skin Deep, Environmental Working Group, accessed
     November 2020, http://www.ewg.org/skindeep/ingredient/702867/HOMOSALATE/; "Octinoxate,"
     EWG's Skin Deep, Environmental Working Group, accessed November 2020, https://www.ewg
     .org/skindeep/ingredients/704203-OCTINOXATE/; Robert Sanders, "Lotion Ingredient Paraben
     May Be More Potent Carcinogen than Thought," *Berkeley News,* UC Berkeley, October 27, 2015,
     https://news.berkeley.edu/2015/10/27/lotion-ingredient-paraben-may-be-more-potent-carcinogen
     -than-thought/.

Chapter 9. Reading Cosmetic Labels, Expiration Dates, and the Slightly Greener Cleanout

1   *allergies and eczema:* Wenyu Liu et. al., "Parabens Exposure in Early Pregnancy and Gestational
     Diabetes Mellitus," *Environment International* 126 (May 2019): 468–475, accessed via PubMed,
     https://pubmed.ncbi.nlm.nih.gov/30844582/; Erika S. Koeppe et. al., "Relationship between
     Urinary Tricolosan and Paraben Concentrations and Serum Thyroid Measures In NHANES
     2007–2008," *The Science of the Total Environment* (February 2013): 299–305, accessed via PubMed,
     https://pubmed.ncbi.nlm.nih.gov/23340023/; Medina S. Jackson-Browne et. al., "The Impact
     of Early-Life Exposure to Antimicrobials on Asthma and Eczema Risk in Children," *Current*
     Environmental Health Reports 6, no.4 (2019): 214–224, https://www.ncbi.nlm.nih.gov/pmc
     /articles/PMC6923583/.

2   *be thrown away:* "Women's Beauty Habits Exposed by NEW Stowaway Cosmetics Survey,"

Stowaway Cosmetics, September 28, 2015, via Cision PR Newswire, https://www.prnewswire.com /news-releases/womens-beauty-habits-exposed-by-new-stowaway-cosmetics-survey-300149858.html.

3   *finish all their makeup:* Alexander Kunst, "Frequency of Makeup Use among U.S. Consumers 2017, by Age," *Statista*, December 20, 2019, https://www.statista.com/statistics/713178/makeup -use-frequency-by-age/.

4   *and higher temperature:* C. Lv et. al., "Investigation on Formaldehyde Release from Preservatives in Cosmetics," *International Journal of Cosmetic Science* 37, no. 5 (October 2015): 474–8, accessed via PubMed, https://www.ncbi.nlm.nih.gov/pubmed/25704726.

5   *"on their labels":* "Shelf Life and Expiration Dating of Cosmetics," U.S. Food & Drug Administration, August 24, 2020, https://www.fda.gov/cosmetics/labeling/expirationdating/default.htm.

6   *every three months:* Dan Gudgel, "How To Use Cosmetics Safely Around Your Eyes," American Academy of Ophthalmology, December 5, 2019, https://www.aao.org/eye-health/tips-pre vention/eye-makeup.

Chapter 10. What's Hiding in Cleaning Supplies, Dust, and Indoor Air

1   *throughout early childhood:* A. Sherrif et. al., "Frequent use of Chemical Household Products Is Associated with Persistent Wheezing in Pre-School Age Children," *Thorax* 60, no. 1 (January 2005): 45–9, accessed via PubMed, https://www.ncbi.nlm.nih.gov/pubmed/15618582.

2   *as other workers:* Jan-Paul Zock et. al., "Update on Asthma and Cleaners," *Current Opinion in Allergy and Clinical Immunology* 10, no. 2 (April 2010): 114–120, accessed via U.S. National Library of Medicine, https://www.ncbi.nlm.nih.gov/pmc/articles/PMC3125175/.

3   *poison control centers:* Institute Staff, "72,947 Calls to Poison Control—The Culprit? Liquid Laundry Pods," Institute for Childhood Preparedness, July 3, 2019, https://www .childhoodpreparedness.org/post/72–947-calls-to-poison-control.

4   *history of dementia:* "Laundry Pods Still a Serious Safety Risk for Kids and People with Dementia, Study Warns," *CBS News,* June 4, 2019, https://www.cbsnews.com/news/laundry-pods-still-a -serious-safety-risk-for-kids-some-people-with-dementia-study/.

5   *their time indoors:* N. E. Klepeis et. al., "The National Human Activity Patter Survey (NHAPS): A Resource for Assessing Exposure to Environmental Pollutants," *Journal of Exposure Analysis and Environmental Epidemiology* 11, no. 3 (May/June 2001): 231–52, accessed via PubMed, https:// www.ncbi.nlm.nih.gov/pubmed/11477521.

6   *than outdoor air:* "Why Indoor Air Quality is Important to Schools," U.S. Environmental Protection Agency, last updated October 5, 2020, https://www.epa.gov/iaq-schools/why-indoor -air-quality-important-schools.

7   *with contaminated air:* Sumedha M. Joshi, "The Sick Building Syndrome," *Indian Journal of Occupational & Environmental Medicine* 12, no. 2 (August 2008): 61–64, accessed via U.S. National Library of Medicine, https://www.ncbi.nlm.nih.gov/pmc/articles/PMC2796751/.

8   *affect cognitive function:* "Green Office Environments Linked with Higher Cognitive Function Scores," Harvard T. H. Chan School of Public Health, October 26, 2015, https://www.hsph .harvard.edu/news/press-releases/green-office-environments-linked-with-higher-cognitive -function-scores/.

9   *their time indoors:* John Bower, "Indoor Air Pollutants and Toxic Materials," Healthy Housing Reference Manual, Centers for Disease Control and Prevention, last updated October 1, 2009, https://www.cdc.gov/nceh/publications/books/housing/cha05.htm.

10   *on their labels:* Roddy Scheer and Doug Moss, "Corporate Whitewash? Why Do Cleaning Product-Makers Keep Most of Their Ingredients Secret?" *Scientific American,* April 13, 2011, https://www.scientificamerican.com/article/toxic-ingredients-cleaning-products/.

11   *and during storms:* Elaine K. Luo, "The Effect of Negative Ions," *Healthline,* September 11, 2019, https://www.healthline.com/health/negative-ions#benefits.

12   *put a salt lamp:* Denise Mann, "Negative Ions Create Positive Vibes," *WebMD,* May 6, 2002, https://www.webmd.com/balance/features/negative-ions-create-positive-vibes#1.

13   *to attract water:* Anne Marie Helmenstine, "Hygroscopic Definition in Chemistry," *ThoughtCo,* December 8, 2019, https://www.thoughtco.com/definition-of-hygroscopic-605230.

14   *bacteria, and viruses:* "Do Himalayan Salt Lamps Really Work?", Negative Ionizers, accessed November 2020, https://negativeionizers.net/himalayan-salt-lamp-benefits-do-salt-lamps -really-work.

15   *in high-humidity environments:* Marina Turea, "Himalayan Salt Lamps: Health Benefits and Buyer's Guide," *Healthcare Weekly,* April 20, 2020, https://healthcareweekly.com/himalayan-salt -lamps/.

16   *depression-relieving qualities:* Hajra Naz and Darakhshan J. Haleem, "Exposure to illuminated salt lamp increases 5-HT metabolism: A serotonergic perspective to its beneficial effects," *Pakistan Journal of Biochemistry & Molecular Biology* 43, no. 2 (2010): 105–108, http://www.pjbmb.org.pk /images/PJBMBArchive/2010/PJBMB_43_2_Jun_2010/13.pdf.

17   *suffer from depression:* Rob Edwards, "Far from Fragrant," *NewScientist,* September 4, 1999, https://www.newscientist.com/article/mg16322022-700-far-from-fragrant/.

18   *inhaling deadly fumes:* Taro Shimizu et. al., "Polymer Fume Fever," *BMJ Case Reports* (2012): bcr2012007790, https://www.ncbi.nlm.nih.gov/pmc/articles/PMC4544973/.

19   *through the oven's vents:* "4 Reasons to Avoid Your Self-Cleaning Oven Feature," Compact Appliance, June 8, 2015, https://learn.compactappliance.com/self-cleaning-oven-hazards/.

20   *"petroleum gases":* "Old English Furniture Polish, Lemon," EWG's Guide to Healthy Cleaning, Environmental Working Group, September 10, 2012, https://www.ewg.org/guides/cleaners/3017 -OLDENGLISHFurniturePolishLemon/.

Chapter 11. When in Doubt, Do It Yourself

1   *harm to the lungs:* Jo-Yu Chin et. al., "Concentrations and Risks of p-Dichlorobenzene in Indoor and Outdoor Air," *Indoor Air* 23, no.1 (February 2013): 40–49, accessed via U.S. National Library of Medicine, https://www.ncbi.nlm.nih.gov/pmc/articles/PMC3501547/.

2   *and general morbidity:* "1,4-Dichlorobenzene (para-Dichlorobenzene): Hazard Summary," U.S. Environmental Protection Agency, January 2000, https://www.epa.gov/sites/production/files/2016–09/documents/1–4-dichlorobenzene.pdf.

3   *lift dirt off surfaces:* Alexandra Ossola, "Why Is Baking Soda Such a Good Cleaner?", *Kitchn,* October 6, 2016, https://www.thekitchn.com/why-is-baking-soda-such-a-good-cleaner-236104.

4   *(or more):* Heidi Nickerson, "How Much Money Does an Average Family Spend on Cleaning Products in a Year?", *The Nest,* June 30, 2018, https://budgeting.thenest.com/much-money-average-family-spend-cleaning-products-year-23539.html.

5   *and reduce headaches:* Helen West, "What Are Essential Oils, and Do They Work?", *Healthline,* September 30, 2019, https://www.healthline.com/nutrition/what-are-essential-oils.

6   *list of disinfectants:* "Force of Nature Disinfecting, Sanitizing & 3rd Party Lab Test Results," Force of Nature, from "Turi Testing Reports, October 2016" Industry Standard Spectrometry Test Results, accessed November 2020, https://www.forceofnatureclean.com/lp-cleaning-disinfecting-test-results/.

7   *noted on the label:* Tara Parker-Pope, "Have I Been Cleaning All Wrong?", *The New York Times,* May 6, 2020, https://www.nytimes.com/2020/05/06/well/live/coronavirus-cleaning-cleaners-disinfectants-home.html.

8   *on porous materials:* Gerardo U. Lopez, "Transfer Efficiency of Bacteria and Viruses from Porous and Nonporous Fomites to Fingers under Different Relative Humidity Conditions," *Applied and Environmental Microbiology* 79, no. 18 (2013): 5728–34, accessed via U.S. National Library of Medicine, https://www.ncbi.nlm.nih.gov/pmc/articles/PMC3754157/.

9   *after twenty-four hours:* "How Long Do Six Common Bacteria and Viruses Last outside the Body?", *Ideal Response,* February 26, 2019, https://www.idealresponse.co.uk/blog/how-long-do-6-common-bacteria-and-viruses-last-outside-the-body/.

10 *viruses and bacteria:* "Boil Water: Technical Brief," World Health Organization, updated January 2015, https://www.who.int/water_sanitation_health/dwq/Boiling_water_01_15.pdf.

11 *damp indoor space:* Y Li et. al., "Role of Ventilation in Airborne Transmission of Infectious Agents in the Built Environment—a Multidisciplinary Systematic Review," *Indoor Air* 17, no. 1 (February 2017): 2–18, accessed via PubMed, https://pubmed.ncbi.nlm.nih.gov/17257148/.

Chapter 12. The Two-Step Cleaning Product Toss

1   *within twenty-four hours:* "Plants Clean Air and Water for Indoor Environments," NASA Technology Transfer Program, 2007, https://spinoff.nasa.gov/Spinoff2007/ps_3.html.

2   *and reduce stress:* Min-sun Lee et. al., "Interaction with Indoor Plants May Reduce Psychological

and Physiological Stress by Suppressing Autonomic Nervous System Activity in Young Adults: A Randomized Cross-over Study," *Journal of Physiological Anthropology* 34, no. 1 (2015): 21, accessed via U.S. National Library of Medicine, https://www.ncbi.nlm.nih.gov/pmc/articles /PMC4419447/; Noma Nazish, "Think You Don't Need Houseplants? Science Says Different," *Forbes*, February 10, 2018, https://www.forbes.com/sites/nomanazish/2018/02/10/think-you -dont-need-houseplants-science-says-different/#751c04e33595.

Appendix A. Resources

1   *cancer-causing asbestos:* Nathan Bomey, "Johnson & Johnson recalls baby powder after discovering small amounts of asbestos," *USA Today*, October 18, 2019, https://www.usatoday.com/story /money/2019/10/18/johnson-johnson-baby-powder-recall-asbestos/4020698002/.

Index

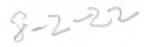

8-2-22

About the Author

Tonya Harris is an award-winning environmental toxin expert and the founder of Slightly Greener, offering busy women simple solutions to reduce toxins in their home without turning their lifestyle upside-down.

As a childhood leukemia survivor and mother of three, Tonya helps parents learn how toxins in the home can affect their family's health. She enjoys helping families detoxify their homes through simple steps, without the overwhelming feeling that commonly comes with it. In addition to a board certification and master's degree in holistic nutrition, she holds multiple certificates in the environmental health field.

Tonya has been featured in *Parents*, *Reader's Digest*, Business Insider, mindbodygreen, and *Martha Stewart Living*, and has appeared on TV shows across the country, such as *Great Day Washington*, *Good Day Charlotte*, CBS New York, KTLA, *Good Day DC*, and *The Dr. Oz Show*, for her expertise in environmental toxins and how toxins affect children.